Eileen R Chadwick

End-of-Life Ethics
and the Nursing Assistant

Eileen R. Chichin, PhD, RN, is the Co-Director of the Center on Ethics at The Jewish Home and Hospital of New York, and an Adjunct Assistant Professor in the Department of Geriatrics and Adult Development of the Mount Sinai School of Medicine. Previously, she was the Assistant Director of the Brookdale Research Institute of the Third Age Center at Fordham University. Dr. Chichin's research and practice interests are in the areas of ethics and end-of-life care for the frail elderly. Her prior publications have focused on ethical issues in the long term care setting.

Orah R. Burack, MA, received her Master of Arts in Psychology from Brandeis University in 1993. After completing requirements for her advanced degree, she received additional training and was involved in several Department of Psychology research projects at Brandeis. This work has been disseminated via presentations at professional conferences and publication in peer-reviewed journals. Since 1996, Ms. Burack has served as the Project Coordinator for a number of research studies undertaken by The Jewish Home and Hospital, focusing primarily on end-of-life ethics and palliative care.

Ellen Olson, MD, is a geriatrician who has been involved in medical ethics since 1987, when she served as a member of the Hastings Center project that resulted in the publication of Guidelines on the *Termination of Life-Sustaining Treatment and the Care of the Dying*. She served as Co-Director of the Kathy and Alan C. Greenberg Center on Ethics and Long-term Care from 1991 until 1998, when she became the Chief of Geriatric Programs at the Bronx Veterans Administration Medical Center in the Bronx, NY. She is also an Associate Professor in the Department of Geriatrics and Adult Development of the Mount Sinai School of Medicine.

Antonios Likourezos, MA, MPH, has a Master of Arts degree in Medical Anthropology from Case Western Reserve University and a Master of Public Health from Columbia University School of Public Health. He is currently a Research Associate at The Jewish Home and Hospital, and holds a faculty appointment in the Department of Geriatrics and Adult Development of the Mount Sinai School of Medicine. His primary interests include research, preventive medicine, and public health policy as it relates to our elderly population.

End-of-Life Ethics and the Nursing Assistant

Eileen R. Chichin, PhD, RN
Orah R. Burack, MA
Ellen Olson, MD
Antonios Likourezos, MA, MPH

 Springer Publishing Company

Springer Publishing Company, Inc.
536 Broadway
New York, NY 10012-3955

Acquisitions Editor: Helvi Gold
Production Editor: Helen Song
Cover design by James Scotto-Lavino

00 01 02 03 04 / 5 4 3 2 1

Library of Congress Cataloging-in-Publication Data

End-of-life ethics and the nursing assistant : and accompanying workbook / Eileen R. Chichin ... [et al.].
    p. cm.
  Includes bibliographical references.
  ISBN 0-8261-1307-9 (hc.)
  1. Terminal care—Moral and ethical aspects. 2. Nurses' aides. 3. Nursing.
I. Chichin, Eileen R.
RT87.T45 E54 2000
174'.24—dc21
                                                99-054061
                                                    CIP

Printed in the United States of America

This book is dedicated to the certified nursing assistants of The Jewish Home and Hospital of New York: our colleagues, our teachers, our friends.

Contents

Foreword

This book and the accompanying workbook deal with the often neglected impact that certified nursing assistants can have on the quality of dying of residents in nursing homes. Whether at home or in a long term care institution, the majority of older Americans now die from the consequences of a chronic illness. While loving family, professional nursing, and medical and therapy staff oversee the care required by people with chronic illness, the actual day-to-day care is most frequently delivered by nursing assistants. As caregiving extends over weeks, months, and sometimes years, as one would expect, nursing assistants, who are primarily women, become emotionally attached to the patient. Thus it should come as no surprise that nursing assistants would have strong feelings and opinions about the dying process for the patients under their care: how the process of dying should proceed; what life-sustaining treatments are and are not appropriate to use; and where and under what circumstances death should occur. Yet, society's newly piqued interest in death and dying rarely reaches down to involve these non-professional caregivers as integral to designing and delivering quality end-of-life care.

The focus of the work reported in this book is on the role of nursing assistants in nursing homes. Nursing homes are increasingly being used as a source of health care for the elderly with acute and chronic illness, and as health care institutions that deliver end-of-life care. Whether on a temporary basis or as a permanent resident, many adults, perhaps as many as a third, who reach an old age or who sustain an acute or chronic illness will spend some time in a nursing facility. A person typically enters a nursing home at a time of great personal vulnerability. Often the person has recently sustained an acute illness that has left them with a deficit—a stroke that has caused residual permanent deficits or a hip fracture that temporarily limits a person's ability to care for herself. At other times, a move to a nursing home results when a chronic illness has progressed to a point where the individual and her family members are unable to continue to manage a care plan at home, for example for persons with dementia, Parkinson's disease, or progressive cancer. The course of these conditions is progressive debility eventually causing the patient's death.

Over the past ten years, rather than transferring dying residents to hospitals, a substantial number of nursing homes have chosen to maintain dying residents within the home. In 1998, 20% of all deaths nationally occurred in nursing homes. The introduction of hospice services in nursing homes and development of protocol for assessment and management of pain attest to the growing interest in establishing best practices in end-of-life care in nursing homes.

The focus of professional educational materials and research aimed at improving end-of-life care in nursing homes has been on upgrading the skills of the professional staff regarding how to assess residents and how to deliver state-of-the-art pain and comfort care. A small body of literature also addresses the need to educate residents and family members as to what to expect in end-of-life care in nursing homes and why remaining in the nursing home during the dying process may be preferable to being transferred to a hospital.

In contrast to professional staff, very little attention has been paid to the involvement and needs of a nursing home's non-professional nursing personnel, specifically certified nursing assistants (CNAs), in creating programs to maintain dying residents within the nursing home. One has only to examine nurse staffing in nursing homes to appreciate the importance of CNAs in the day-to-day delivery of care to residents. Typically, in nursing homes, certified nursing assistants deliver most of the care. Staffing in nursing homes is such that, in an average home, there will be a professional Registered Nurse (RN) as Director of Nursing, who is in the home during the day, perhaps a second RN in the home during the day shift, and a licensed practical nurse (LPN) in charge on evenings and at night. The majority of the direct care of nursing home residents falls to the certified nursing assistants (CNAs), non-professional nursing personnel who have received minimum on the job training and who work for minimum wage. While turnover of CNAs is notoriously high, an average of 100% annually in many nursing homes, CNAs are loyal employees who have worked as nursing assistants and particularly in nursing homes over many years. Thus many CNAs have long-standing relationships with residents. For some residents, the CNA assumes the role of surrogate family member.

The importance of CNAs in the delivery of end-of-life care in nursing homes and the paucity of knowledge as to how CNAs feel about this care is the background for the work reported by Chichin and her colleagues in this volume. The work reported here is unique and groundbreaking in its approach to improving end-of-life care in nursing homes. First, it focuses on learning directly from CNAs how they perceive the care that they deliver to dying residents. As described in the introduction and overview of the book, the overall goal was to determine CNAs' knowledge, attitudes, and feelings about ethical issues and end-of-life decision making. The implication is that there is something to be learned from CNAs about how to structure quality end-of-life care. Secondly, the volume focuses on strategies that nursing homes can use to support CNAs in their care of dying residents. Particularly noteworthy are the focus on educational programs to increase CNA knowledge about end-of-life care, incorporation of strategies that CNAs can use to improve comfort care, and the creation of support groups that focus on the needs of CNAs as they care for increasing numbers of dying residents.

The findings, analysis, and recommendations that emanate from this book and workbook are cause for reflection on how best to structure end-of-life care in nursing homes. The book offers insight to professional personnel in nursing homes, nurses, physicians, and social workers, on how CNAs feel about the care they are asked to deliver, CNAs' frustrations with their relative lack of involvement in that care, and the needs that CNAs have if they are to sustain caregiving activities with dying residents. These insights should lead professional care providers to improve the education and involvement of CNAs in the team process of health care delivery. For nursing home administrators, the findings reported in this book should suggest strategies that need to be in place to train and keep CNAs at the bedside. The accompanying workbook will facilitate implementing an educational program in any nursing home facility.

The text raises cautionary flags for agencies that oversee policy, regulation and reimbursement for nursing homes. Reimbursement procedures for care in nursing homes must take into account the added resources that homes need to adequately care for dying residents. If the public is to have confidence in the end-of-life care delivered in nursing homes, federal and state regulations need to require homes to have professional nursing and medical staff, and non-professional nursing staff, with the knowledge and skills and present in sufficient number to deliver quality care to dying residents. The work of Chichin, Burack, Olson, and Likourezos reminds us that involving CNAs is a fruitful and essential step to be taken if residents in nursing homes are to die in the home with comfort and dignity.

Mathy D. Mezey, EdD, RN, FAAN
Independence Foundation Professor of Nursing Education and
Director, the Hartford Institute for Geriatric Nursing Education
Division of Nursing
New York University
New York, NY

1

Introduction and Overview

Advances in medical technology are allowing our society to keep people alive far longer than ever before. This is perhaps most evident in nursing homes, where frail elderly may live for many years with conditions that cause profound cognitive impairment and physical decline. And, while a common sequela of these disorders often renders its victims unable to swallow, the use of life-sustaining treatment such as artificial nutrition and hydration can prolong their lives for many years. Many individuals question whether they would like their own lives extended in such cases and in such a fashion. Since the passage of the federal Patient Self Determination Act in 1991, all people have been assured of our prerogative to limit such treatment. An increase in national awareness of our individual right to make decisions about health care, including the refusal of life-sustaining treatment, has caused a rise in the number of people who execute advance directives limiting the use of artificial nutrition and hydration in certain cases.

Respecting a person's right to limit life-sustaining treatment often has a marked impact on health care providers, especially those who work in nursing homes. Of particular note is the effect of treatment termination on certified nursing assistants (CNAs). These individuals provide the bulk of hands-on care in long term care facilities and develop close relationships with the residents for whom they care. Often, they are assigned to the same residents for a period of years, during which they provide the most intimate aspects of physical care. Additionally, in many instances, they are the primary providers of emotional support to nursing home residents. In fact, they may often become surrogate family members to the residents for whom they care. Accordingly, when residents opt to have life-sustaining treatment withheld or withdrawn, the CNAs are profoundly affected.

Professional staff in nursing homes may also have strong feelings about caring for residents who opt to have life-sustaining treatment limited. However, professionals have the opportunity to educate themselves about these issues, attending conferences and reading journals. Nursing assistants, on the other hand, are generally left out of the educational loop. CNAs may be told that a resident for whom they cared for several years can no longer swallow and will not be receiving a feeding tube. The role of the CNA is to continue to provide care to the resident until the resident dies, but the CNA is generally not asked her or his opinion and is not part of the decision-making process.

The emotional discomfort associated with caring for residents dying without life-sustaining treatment is very likely exacerbated by nursing assistants' limited knowledge of ethical principles related to end-of-life treatment decision-making. Perhaps even more

1

distressing, however, is the perception that they may actually have contributed to the resident's death by not continuing to provide life-sustaining care. The fact that limitation of life-sustaining treatment occurs out of respect for the resident's autonomous choice is usually not recognized by nursing assistants.

Little, if anything, is known about the extent to which CNAs understand these issues, as well as how they feel about caring for residents who opt to limit life-sustaining treatment. Thus, with the generous support of the Greenwall Foundation, the current project was undertaken to remedy this situation. Its goals were:

to determine how knowledgeable nursing assistants, employed in long term care, are about ethical issues and end-of-life decision-making.

to assess nursing assistants' attitudes about ethical issues at the end of life.

to develop a replicable program to provide support to nursing assistants and educate them about ethical issues, treatment decision-making, and comfort care at the end of life.

to determine whether participation in such a program influences knowledge and attitudes about ethics.

The following review of the literature describes what is known about ethics education for health care workers in general, as well as recommendations for CNAs. The role of the nursing assistant in the care of nursing home residents will also be described. This will set the stage for a detailed description of the methodology and findings drawn from this project.

WHAT THE LITERATURE TELLS US

In order to raise the awareness of health care providers regarding the rights of patients to make treatment decisions, a number of nursing homes and hospitals nationwide implemented ethics education programs. Perhaps the most notable of these programs is Decisions Near the End of Life, developed by the Education Development Center in Newton, Massachusetts, and the Hastings Center in Garrison, NY (Solomon et al., 1991). This excellent program provides a broad education in end-of-life decision-making for professionals in hospitals and nursing homes. However, it does not address the needs of paraprofessional staff. This is problematic for health care providers in nursing homes since they play such a significant role—a role that has been noted in the long term care literature (Bowers & Becker, 1992; Collopy, Boyle, & Jennings, 1991; Foner, 1994; Libow & Starer, 1989; Looman, Noelker, Schur, Whitlatch, & Ejaz, 1997). As noted earlier, these workers deliver the bulk of "hands-on" care to the frail elderly who reside in nursing homes (Aroskar, Urv-Wong, & Kane, 1990). Included among the many tasks they perform are bathing, toileting, feeding, and providing companionship to dependent older persons. Often, as noted earlier, the intimacy, closeness, and longevity of the interactions that occur between these two members of the caregiving dyad cause these workers to become, in effect, surrogate family to their nursing home residents. In fact, it is a paraprofessional staff member who frequently becomes the single most important person in the daily life of the nursing home resident.

In general, literature focusing on ethics education for health care staff has been relatively minimal. And, although the need for programs to address the needs of nursing assistants has been emphasized (Olson et al., 1992), as mentioned above, programs undertaken to date have been limited to those addressing the needs of professional staff only (Olson et al., 1992; Solomon et al., 1991). This literature does suggest that ethics education seems to be a most effective route toward assisting health care providers at all levels to make optimum health care decisions, and consequently deliver the highest level of care to critically or terminally ill individuals.

In addition to the paucity of literature on ethics education, there has been minimal attention paid to the needs of nursing home staff who care for the dying, with the exception of the work of Linn, Linn, and Stein (1983). Their findings suggest that educating nursing home staff about death and dying enhances their ability to care for both dying residents and their families. The majority of research on health care providers who regularly care for dying patients has been drawn primarily from the realm of hospice care and has not focused on the long term care setting. This literature suggests that care givers frequently experience grief reactions (Benoliel, 1974; Lerea & LiMauro, 1982; Lev, 1989), and numerous other emotional difficulties (Harper, 1977; Kastenbaum, 1967; Koocher, 1979; Rando, 1984; Strauss, 1968).

It seems likely that much of this hospice literature is generalizable to those working in nursing homes. Nursing home staff also regularly care for the dying, although usually over a far longer period of time, since a number of nursing home stays are of several years' duration. And increasingly, nursing home residents are dying because they have exercised their right to autonomy and have opted not to have life-sustaining treatment. Thus, while it may be difficult for caregiving staff in nursing homes when their residents die, it may be even more painful when the death is a result of the resident's autonomous choice. It seems to follow, then, that a program that incorporates not only education about ethics, but also allows participants to share their concerns about these issues and be supported, would be most effective.

Two prior studies undertaken by the Center on Ethics at The Jewish Home and Hospital of New York (Chichin, 1995; Chichin, Schulman, Harrington, Norwood, & Olson, 1995), as well as a third study (Chichin & Olson, 1998) conducted contemporaneously with the current Greenwall Foundation study, support the need to involve CNAs in ethics education in nursing homes. In one study (Chichin et al., 1995), we surveyed 250 of our own nursing assistants in The Jewish Home to determine their knowledge and attitudes about ethical issues related to life-sustaining treatment. In another study piloting a survey of the impact on staff of caregiving in treatment termination situations (Chichin, 1995), we interviewed ten nursing assistants who had cared for residents who had died as a result of treatment termination.

In the first project, assessing CNAs' knowledge and attitudes about ethical issues and end-of-life decision-making, we found a relatively high level of knowledge about facility policies related to these issues, as well as knowledge about many ethical issues in general. Also surprising was the extent to which the responses of the CNAs mirrored those of our professional staff who completed a similar questionnaire when the Decisions program was conducted at The Jewish Home. However, we suspect that our population of nursing assistants in a large, urban teaching nursing home with a ten-year history of work in the field of ethics may not be representative of nursing assistants in other settings.

In the second and third studies (Chichin, 1995; Chichin & Olson, 1998), qualitative interviews with CNAs revealed they have very strong feelings about care of the dying and treatment termination, and often do not feel supported in their work. In general, our experience with both these studies and our work to date with nursing assistants suggested strongly that they need a sound educational foundation in ethical principles, particularly respect for autonomy. This is necessary to help them accept, on both an intellectual and emotional level, the autonomous choices of the residents for whom they care. Additionally, education in ethics and end-of-life decision-making has also been recommended by others closely involved in research with CNAs (Looman et al., 1997), and should help CNAs carry out the difficult tasks associated with providing care to residents who opt to have life-sustaining treatment withheld or withdrawn.

This book describes the project that was developed to assess CNAs' knowledge and attitudes about ethical issues and end-of-life decision-making, as well as the educational intervention and support group program that were designed to meet their needs. Accompanying this volume is a workbook that will enable other nursing facilities to implement the program on their own.

The project focused on three main areas: the role of the nursing assistant in the end-of-life care of nursing home residents, the principle of respect for autonomy, and the use of comfort care. To put our findings in context, three of the chapters of this book will give an overview of each of these respective areas. Following this introductory chapter, chapter 2 focuses on what is generally known about CNAs, drawn both from research and from our anecdotal experience with them. This chapter also discusses how CNAs feel about their work, how they feel about their residents, and what nursing homes can do to support them as they provide care to some of the frailest members of our society.

In chapter 3, the principle of respect for autonomy is discussed, with attention paid to issues that may influence how CNAs feel about this principle. Chapter 4 is an overview of comfort care, with an emphasis on the role of CNAs in providing these most important components of care at the end of life.

Chapters 5 and 6 cover the study methods and findings, respectively. The next three chapters are a discussion of the findings, with chapter 7 focusing on CNAs, how they view themselves, and how we view them. In chapter 8, we look at what the CNAs in this project knew and felt about issues related to respecting resident autonomy, and chapter 9 is an overview of how the CNAs felt about delivering comfort care, and again emphasizing the important role that CNAs can play here.

We were particularly interested in learning how CNAs felt about the project. Chapter 10, therefore, includes a detailed overview of the CNAs' evaluation of the educational program.

In a separate component of the project, we developed support groups whose focus was to provide an environment in which CNAs could feel comfortable discussing their concerns around care of the dying, and receive emotional support in the process. Chapter 11 describes this support group program in detail

In chapter 12, we discuss what we see as the implications of our findings, and what nursing homes can do to educate and support CNAs as they carry out their important work.

Conducting this project was an extremely interesting and challenging experience. It reinforced to us the importance of the role played by CNAs. It also gave us the opportunity of getting to know, at least on some level, over 600 nursing assistants. We found this to be both a privilege and a pleasure, and often felt we learned more from them than they learned from us. We hope our nursing home colleagues will undertake this program with similar results. It can only benefit our certified nursing assistants, and by extension, the growing number of nursing home residents for whom we all share responsibility.

REFERENCES

Aroskar, M. A., Urv-Wong, E., & Kane, R. A. (1990). Building an effective care-giving staff: Transforming the nursing service. In R. A. Kane & A. L. Caplan (Eds.), *Everyday ethics: Resolving dilemmas in nursing home life* (pp. 271–290). New York: Springer.

Benoliel, J. Q. (1974). Anticipatory grief in physicians and nurses. In B. Schoenberg, A. C. Carr, A. H. Kutscher, D. Peretz, & I. K. Goldberg (Eds.), *Anticipatory grief* (pp. 218–228). New York: Columbia University Press.

Bowers, B., & Becker, M. (1992). Nurse's aides in nursing homes: the relationship between organization and quality. *The Gerontologist, 32*(3), 360–366.

Chichin, E. R. (1995). Treatment termination in long-term care: Implications for health care providers. In E. Olson, E. R. Chichin, & L. S. Libow (Eds.), *Controversies in ethics in long-term care* (pp. 29–42). New York: Springer.

Chichin, E. R., & Olson, E. (1998). Staff reactions to dementia patients' requests to withhold or withdraw treatment. Final Report to the New York State Department of Health Bureau of Long-term Care Services.

Chichin, E. R., Schulman, E., Harrington, M., Norwood, J., & Olson, E. (1995). End-of-life treatment decisions in the nursing home: Ethics and the nursing assistant. In P. Katz, R. Kane, and M. Mezey (Eds.), *Advances in long-term care* (pp. 116–129). New York: Springer.

Collopy, B., Boyle, B., & Jennings, B. (1991). New directions in nursing home ethics. *Hastings Center Report, Special Supplement March-April*, 1–15.

Foner, N. (1994). Nursing home aides: Saints or monsters? *The Gerontologist, 34*(2), 245–250.

Harper, B. (1977). *Death: The coping mechanism of the health professional.* Greenville, SC: Southeastern University Press.

Kastenbaum, R. (1967). Multiple perspectives on a geriatric "Death Valley." *Community Mental Health Journal, 3*, 21–29.

Koocher, G. (1979). Adjustment and coping strategies among the caretakers of cancer patients. *Social Work in Health Care, 5*, 145–151.

Lerea, L. E., & LiMauro, B. F. (1982). Grief among health care workers: A comparative study. *Journal of Gerontology, 37*(5), 604–608.

Lev, E. (1989). A nurse's perspective on disenfranchised grief. In K. Doka (Ed.), *Disenfranchised grief* (pp. 287–299). Lexington, MA: D. C. Heath.

Libow, L. S., & Starer, P. (1989). Care of the nursing home patient. *New England Journal of Medicine, 321*(2), 93–96.

Linn, M. W., Linn, B. S., & Stein, S. (1983). Impact on nursing home staff of training about death and dying. *Journal of the American Medical Association, 250*(17), 2332–2335.

Looman, W. J., Noelker, L. S., Schur, D., Whitlatch, C. J., & Ejaz, F. (1997). Nursing assistants caring for dementia residents in nursing homes: The family's perspective on the high quality of care. *American Journal of Alzheimer's Care*, 221–226.

Olson, E., Martico-Greenfield, T., Carlos, A., Jackson, R., Guilfoy, V., & Jennings, B. (1992). Ethics education in long-term care: The Decisions Near the End of Life program. *Journal of Health Administration Education, 10*(4), 611–622.

Rando, T. (1984). *Grief, dying and death: Clinical interventions for caregivers.* Champaign, IL: Research Press.

Solomon, M. Z., Jennings, B., Guilfoy, V., Jackson, R., O'Donnell, L., Wolf, S., Nolan, K., Koch-Weser, D., & Donnelly, S. (1991). Toward an expanded vision of clinical ethics education: From the individual to the institution. *Kennedy Institute of Ethics Journal, 1*(3), 225–246.

Strauss, A. (1968). The intensive care unit: Its characteristics and social relationships. *Nursing Clinics of North America, 3*, 7–15.

2

The Certified Nursing Assistant

In the nursing home world, certified nursing assistants (CNAs) play a lead role, particularly in the lives of those who live there. Although they are generally among the least educated and least skilled workers (Collopy, Boyle, & Jennings, 1991), they form the foundation of the nursing home staff. Viewed as a pyramid, staffing in nursing homes has paraprofessional and non-professional personnel (such as nursing assistants, food service workers, and housekeeping staff) forming the base of the pyramid, and professional staff (i.e., administrators, registered nurses, and social workers) forming the upper parts of the structure. In most nursing homes, the professional component of the staff is significantly smaller than the para- and non-professional component. However, in every nursing home, the nursing assistant provides the bulk of hands-on care to nursing home residents, and generally becomes the most important person in the everyday life of the nursing home resident.

Many CNAs are drawn from the same personnel pool as those individuals who work in the fast food industry. As Garland and his colleagues (Garland, Oyabu, & Gipson, 1988) tell us, CNAs tend to be women, and often are single parents. Most have a high school education or less. And, while incomes vary, many, especially those who are not unionized, tend to be paid minimum wage. Many come from minority backgrounds, and, as noted above, in general are relatively unskilled individuals. In numerous cases, certain characteristics of CNAs (e.g., age, gender, level of education, and ethnic background) limit their employment opportunities. Poorly paid, minimally trained, and overworked (Collopy et al., 1991), many CNAs tend not to stay in the same nursing home or even in the field for a very long time. Turnover in the industry has been estimated at 40 to 70 percent nationwide (Waxman, Carner, & Berkenstock, 1984), although a number do stay for longer periods. Those who tend to remain employed in the field for longer periods of time often do so because they believe they have job security. Additionally, they appreciate many of what they see as the intrinsic rewards of the job. Most prominent among these intrinsic rewards is the ability to form close emotional relationships with those residents assigned to their care in the nursing home (Garland et al., 1988). While some research suggests that many CNAs are "curt, condescending and cruel" (Fontana, 1977; Gubrium, 1975; Kayser-Jones, 1990; Tellis-Nayak & Tellis-Nayak, 1989), many CNAs define themselves "as nurturing, caring, and compassionate people who help the sick. (Some see their role) as a religious calling or mission" (Heiselman & Noelker, 1991, p. 554).

In conducting in-depth interviews with CNAs (Chichin & Olson, 1997), we found many of the nursing assistants deeply committed to their work. Some examples of their statements include the following:

(My work) is meaningful . . . (and) I love to do it and I love the residents assigned to me. The care I give them is the same care I would give if it were my own mother or father. It's not 40 or 60 per cent; it's 100 percent. I do this because I want to. I don't do this because I want praise.

What I try to do is, if I see somebody who I know is not going to be here long, I go into their room and if they are unresponsive I try to hold their hand for a while and let them know somebody is there, and I know what is going on. If they're responsive and alert, I sit down and talk to them for a while to be a friend so that they can have somebody and they don't feel that they are by themselves . . . I let them feel there is somebody there.

I get satisfaction (from this work). I know that I bring residents comfort through myself. I know how I want to handle them as far as giving them an extra backrub, saying a prayer with them (even though many of them are a different religion than I am). I know I can comfort them just by being there.

We're like a family (to the residents). We're there eight hours a day, five days a week and I think at times I feel the staff is more attached than the family.

Last week one of my residents went into a relapse and we thought she was dying and we went berserk. You would have thought we were the EMS trying to bring her back to life. I started to cry because I love her so dearly.

In conducting the Greenwall Foundation study on which this book is based, we did encounter a few CNAs who denied feeling emotionally close to residents. They claimed they provided the same care to everyone, and did not form close attachments. The majority of CNAs in the study, however, strongly believed this was not realistic. Furthermore, they felt they could provide better care to the residents assigned to them if they did develop close relationships. They felt this enabled them to see each resident as an individual, and thus provide individualized care to the maximum extent possible given the constraints of time and a large assignment. Most also agreed they had certain residents who became favorites and with whom they formed even closer relationships.

While we suspect that most CNAs are compassionate, caring individuals, clearly there may be some who do not fit this mold. Foner's (1994) work with CNAs in a nursing home in New York City found them to be "neither saints nor monsters." Rather, she described only a very small group who she could characterize as "consistently cruel" (p. 245), while a similar minority were consistently warm and supportive. Foner saw some losing their tempers, and behaving in ways that perhaps would appear to be mean to someone unfamiliar with the situation. She found that most CNAs, most of the time, were kind and helpful to those for whom they care. Particularly noteworthy about this is the fact that they maintained primarily positive behaviors in the face of overwhelming physical and emotional demands, and often when they were actually physically abused by residents.

EXACTLY WHAT DO CNAS DO?

The "work world" of the certified nursing assistant, the long term care institution, is the final home for many of the oldest and frailest individuals in this country. Most nursing homes are for-profit enterprises, with only about one-quarter having not-for-profit status. Most have fewer than 100 beds (Strahan, 1987), although many facilities in New York State (one of the states where the project was conducted) are significantly larger. New York State nursing homes are also more likely than facilities in the rest of the country to be not-for-profit. Nationwide, these beds are generally filled with widowed white women (Hing, 1989), most of whose care is provided for by Medicaid (Foner, 1994).

In the nursing home, certified nursing assistants perform 80 to 100 percent of the hands-on care (Institute of Medicine, 1986). This "bed and body" work (Gubrium, 1975) consists of such time-intensive and physically challenging tasks as bathing, toileting, feeding, positioning, and transferring from bed to chair. As Foner (1994) describes it, the work of the nursing assistant involves "taking (residents) to the bathroom, offering a bedpan, or most often, changing their incontinent briefs. Bedfast patients must be turned and positioned every two hours. There is regular paperwork too, such as recording vital signs and regular bowel movements" (p. 247). As well, CNAs must perform certain assessments, such as monitoring temperature, pulse and respiration. Unfortunately, CNAs are "often incorrectly viewed as the ones who clean up incontinent residents, clean up vomit and generally just clean up" (Aroskar, Urv-wong, & Kane, 1990, p. 275). While these tasks are clearly part of their job description, every nursing assistant accomplishes far more than just those tasks.

Perhaps most important to nursing home residents and their families, CNAs often form strong emotional attachments with the residents for whom they care. CNAs become, in many instances, surrogate family members to their nursing home residents. Some CNAs have described situations to us in which the resident seems to feel so close to the nursing assistant that when the family arrives, the resident is reluctant to interact with the family, preferring instead to remain with the nursing assistant. This, of course, is usually quite distressing to the family member. Nonetheless, to the nursing assistant, the formation of relationships with residents is the most satisfying aspect of the work they do. As Aroskar and her colleagues (1990) remind us, these relationships develop even when, as is almost always the case, CNAs and the residents for whom they care generally have different backgrounds. Even when the nursing assistant is carrying a massive workload, she usually finds time for the emotional aspects of the job.

And indeed, the workload of the nursing assistant is generally rather large. CNAs are usually assigned about eight to ten residents, depending on the level of care required by the resident. The level of care can vary markedly, depending upon a resident's cognitive and functional capacity. Some residents may be fairly high-functioning, needing only assistance with some activities of daily living. Others may need help with almost everything, and a few may need every personal task performed for them by the nursing assistant. And, from time to time, a nursing assistant may care for a resident who is actively dying, a situation fraught with its own special emotional issues.

CNAs are responsible for all aspects of care for these residents, an often overwhelming task. How to accomplish this is a daunting task for the nursing assistant. Bowers and Becker (1992), in studying CNAs, found that for many, the primary concern was simply getting the job done. How to do this was often something they had to learn on their own, for while CNAs are taught a variety of tasks and are given a great deal of information when they receive their initial job training, they are not taught how to prioritize. They are often faced with simultaneous demands, but do not know how to cope with being required to accomplish so much all at the same time. Not surprisingly, Bowers and Becker (1992) found a very high proportion of CNAs resigning within a few weeks of being hired because of job responsibilities they had no idea how to handle. Although in much of our work we found CNAs who were employed for many years as nursing assistants, we are not sure the extent to which their lengthy tenure on the job is generalizable across the country.

In our work with the CNAs in the Greenwall Foundation project, they regularly cited a number of situations they found particularly difficult. Early in their careers as CNAs, they find simply adjusting to the nursing home and to the work a challenge and often quite difficult. Over time, as they become very close to certain residents and one of those residents becomes sick and dies it can feel as if a member of the nursing assistant's own family has died. If a resident dies while the nursing assistant is caring for him or her, or immediately after care, CNAs sometimes question whether they may have done something wrong and in some way may have caused the resident's death.

Particularly intense is the first time a resident dies, and caring for the body after death. Often this is the nursing assistant's initial experience with death, and it may be frightening to the nursing assistant. In discussing this with the administrator of a Carmelite facility in rural New York State, she told us of her experience with CNAs caring for the dying for the first time. "You have nothing to fear from those who are dying," she would tell the CNAs. "You have far more to fear from those who are living. When you are caring for the dying, yours is the last face they will see before they stand before the throne of God. They can only do you good" (personal communication, Sr. M. Bernadette Therese, O. Carm., October 4, 1996). Interestingly, this philosophy seemed to be implemented in the facility where she worked at the time she told us this story. There, CNAs told us how they sought out the opportunity to sit at the bedside of dying residents and comfort them.

CNAs also are distressed by difficult work situations. One they described to us involved caring for a resident with gangrene who refused to have an amputation. When it came to certain issues around treatments, particularly the use (or non-use) of life-sustaining treatments such as feeding tubes, it was difficult for the nursing assistant when it was not clear if the treatment decision was based on resident's wishes or the family's request.

OTHER ISSUES IN THE LIVES AND WORK OF THE CERTIFIED NURSING ASSISTANT

A number of personal and professional issues may influence the work lives of nursing assistants, and may serve to either improve or worsen the quality of their work. At the personal level, CNAs may have financial and family issues that strain their abilities to perform at the highest level. As noted earlier, the income level of the nursing assistant may make it very difficult to make ends meet. Many bear the responsibility of child-rearing alone, and have concerns about child care while they themselves are at work. Many may live in areas that are less than safe, and travel to work may be an added burden. The Tellis-Nayaks (1989), in their work on the world of the nursing assistant, suggest that CNAs may have difficulty in performing on the job because of these stressors in their personal lives.

Stressors are also present in the workplace. Simply caring for the cognitively-impaired has been shown to be very burdensome (Chappel & Novak, 1992). In fact, the stress of nursing home work may influence staff, on occasion, to be abusive to residents. And unfortunately, as the work of Pillemer and Moore (1989) suggests, this may be more widespread than we would like to believe.

Brown (1987) describes a highly disturbing situation when discussing the work environment of many CNAs: "they are constantly frustrated, confused, and exasperated when immediately after cleaning and grooming their clients, they hear and see them soiling and disheveling themselves. (They are) assigned patient loads that would make exacting demands upon the physical strength of any two workers. They are at risk to physical injury via provoked or unprovoked attack by resistive clients, e.g., being hit by canes, thrown objects, or bitten severely enough (by even toothless clients) to require medical attention. The use of demeaning epithets and the hurling of various racial slurs seem to 'go with the territory' " (p. 9). As one nursing director told us in the course of our conducting this project, "I'd rather work in a fast food restaurant than be a nursing assistant—they work too hard!"

Despite all this, CNAs view their residents as unique individuals (Bowers, 1988). As noted earlier, they form very strong emotional bonds with their residents. This is clearly a positive thing most of the time, but has a profound impact on the nursing assistant when a resident is dying (Wilson & Daley, 1998). In our Greenwall Foundation project, many CNAs stated they would appreciate some sort of emotional support when caring for dying residents, but, short of empathetic co-workers, this support rarely materialized. In fact, the implicit or explicit feeling was that CNAs were discouraged from becoming attached to residents. Then, when the resident died, there would be no or little sense of bereavement or loss on the part of the nursing assistant. As noted in the workbook accompanying this volume, the message given to CNAs is that they are not supposed to be sad when a resident dies—it's just part of the job.

Interestingly, families note and appreciate the emotional attachments between their institutionalized relative and the nursing assistant (Looman, Noelker, Schur, Whitlatch, & Ejaz, 1997). As well, they are grateful for the care provided by CNAs, and are concerned about understaffing, heavy workloads, and low wages. When Duncan and Morgan (1994) conducted focus groups with families to assess their perceptions of nursing home staff, they found that the family members who participated in their groups had more positive things to say about CNAs than any other staff members in the nursing home. Particularly noteworthy in the work of Duncan and Morgan was that families do not see "technically excellent" care as most important. Rather, "from the family's perspective, caring for (the) resident is not just a set of tasks, but an ongoing process that must occur in meaningful relationships . . . what families seek from nursing homes is . . . the process of caring about the resident" (p. 244).

WHAT CAN BE DONE TO SUPPORT CNAS?

As noted above, the work role of the certified nursing assistant is a difficult one, both physically and emotionally. The financial rewards are minimal, and while some CNAs stay in the job because it is easier than finding other work, many more chose this work and find many aspects of it to be meaningful. CNAs are the primary caregivers of some of the oldest and frailest members of our society. Unfortunately, we as a society have tended to underestimate the value of their work. Perhaps it is time to take another look at how important this work truly is, and what can be done to support those who do it. Undertaking this end-of-life ethics project for nursing assistants enabled us learn a great deal about CNAs and to zero in on a number of areas where we can support them. In addition, there has been some earlier work that has also addressed these issues in a superb fashion.

In Kane and Caplan's (1990) excellent work on "Everyday Ethics" in nursing homes, Aroskar, Urv-Wong, and Kane suggest some concrete solutions. Some similar suggestions are found in the work of Schur, Noelker, Looman, Whitlatch, and Ejaz (1998).

First of all, educational support for nursing assistants needs to be ongoing. More importantly, however, it needs to be meaningful. As Schur and her colleagues (1998) remind us, federal regulations mandate 75 hours of initial training for CNAs, followed by 12 hours every year. This annual training covers topics such as infection control, fire safety, and confidentiality and resident/patient dignity, but generally these topics are presented in such a routinized fashion that they are totally uninteresting to CNAs. Training in areas where CNAs really feel the need for additional education (e.g., dealing with abusive behaviors, care of the dying, and basic human relations skills) tends to be minimal or non-existent.

Aroskar et al. (1990) note that CNAs are taught to make observations. Seldom, however, are they told why these observations are important, and what actions may be taken based on these observations. The degree of accuracy of these observations may be influenced significantly if the nursing assistant understands the rationale behind the observation.

It may be useful to involve CNAs in deciding what topics are the focus of their educational programs. Professional staff, who regularly attend conferences, are routinely asked what they would like to have addressed in future conferences. CNAs are rarely offered the opportunity to request what topics they would like to have covered in in-service situations. Involving CNAs in educational planning can only serve to make the educational sessions more relevant and more appealing to the CNAs. This translates into improved resident care.

CNAs also need to feel they are part of the decision-making and care-planning process, and simply not automatons to whom tasks are delegated. As noted elsewhere, CNAs spend the greatest amount of time with the resident, and generally have the greatest sense of the resident's condition. Ignoring the input of CNAs minimizes the degree to which observations of residents' conditions will be accurate, and subsequently minimizes the chances that interventions will be appropriate. Further, involving CNAs in decisions about resident care gives them a greater investment in the delivery and quality of that care. A serendipitous result is enhancing the CNAs' sense of their importance as members of the health care team.

The quality of supervision provided to CNAs is another area where we might focus our attention (Schur et al., 1998). The study undertaken by Schur and her colleagues found a number of CNAs dissatisfied with the supervisory personnel with whom they dealt. CNAs need supervisors who are skilled in management techniques, who acknowledge the good work of CNAs and recognize the importance of their contributions to resident care. Often the supervisors of nursing assistants in long term care facilities are nurses who do not, as part of their training, receive education in how to oversee the work of other professional and para-professional staff. Schur and her colleagues recommend training supervisors in areas such as conflict management, methods of motivating staff, and delivering constructive feedback. Perhaps most important for these supervisors is learning how to praise sound job performance.

Another area that needs to be addressed when attempting to improve the work life of nursing assistants involves the repeated losses experienced by CNAs caring for dying nursing home residents. Karioth (1998), discussing how to help CNAs deal with grief and bereavement, noted that CNAs "are as much on the front lines as cops, firemen, and rescue workers," but unlike these individuals, are not offered a "debriefing" when someone dies (p. 2). She notes that nursing home staffing is such that CNAs cannot be given time off in which to grieve. However, validating their loss, noting, "this must be hard for you," in combination with short breaks when a nursing assistant feels overwhelmed, can be helpful. Dr. Karioth recommends developing any kinds of rituals that will help in the grieving process. If possible, CNAs should try to go to the funeral home, and optimally, the nursing home should support this by giving extra time off. She also suggests that CNAs write cards to the family, expressing their condolences. CNAs should be educated to the fact that grief is natural and normal, and to be expected when a resident to whom they have become close becomes very ill and dies. Nursing homes, as well, should recognize this fact, and support CNAs who are experiencing the loss of a resident.

Clearly, there are some negatives in the personal and work life of CNAs that we do not have the ability to change. However, there are also a number of issues within our reach that we can and should address. So doing will enhance the ability of CNAs to perform the difficult tasks they face on a daily basis, and ultimately improve the care provided to the frail elderly population in our nation's nursing homes.

REFERENCES

Aroskar, M. A., Urv-Wong, E. K., & Kane, R. A. (1990). Building an effective caregiving staff: Transforming the nursing service. In R. A. Kane & A. L. Caplan (Eds.), *Everyday ethics: Resolving dilemmas in nursing home life* (pp. 271–290). New York: Springer.

Bowers, B. J. (1988). Family perceptions of care in a nursing home. *The Gerontologist, 28*(3), 361–368.

Bowers, B. J., & Becker, M. (1992). Nurses aides in nursing homes: The relationship between organization and quality. *The Gerontologist, 32*(3), 360–366.

Brown, C. T. (1987). An anguished relationship: The white aged institutionalized client and the non-white paraprofessional worker. In R. Dobrof (Ed.), *Ethnicity and gerontological social work* (pp. 3–12). New York: Haworth.

Chappell, N. L., & Novak, M. (1992). The role of support in alleviating stress among nursing assistants. *The Gerontologist, 34*(3), 351–359.

Chichin, E. R., & Olson, E. (1997). Reasons for staff discomfort with dementia patients requests to withhold or withdraw life-sustaining treatment. Final Report. New York State Department of Health Bureau of Long-term Care Services Dementia Grant Project.

Collopy, B., Boyle, P., & Jennings, B. (1991). New directions in nursing home ethics. *Hastings Center Report, Special Supplement March-April,* 1–15.

Duncan, M. T., & Morgan, D. C. (1994). Sharing the caring: Family caregivers views on their relationships with nursing home staff. *The Gerontologist, 34*(2), 234–244.

Foner, N. (1994) Nursing home aides: Saints or monsters? *The Gerontologist, 34*(2), 245–250.

Fontana, A. (1977). *The last frontier.* Beverly Hills, CA: Sage.

Garland, T. N., Oyabu, N., & Gipson, G. A. (1988). Stayers and leavers: A comparison of nursing assistants employed in nursing homes. *Journal of Long-term Care Administration (Winter)*, 23–29.

Gubrium, J. (1975). *Living and dying at Murray Manor*. New York: St. Martin's Press.

Heiselman, T., & Noelker, L. S. (1991). Enhancing mutual respect among nursing assistants, residents, and residents' families. *The Gerontologist, 31*(40), 552–555.

Hing, E. (1989). *Nursing home utilization by current residents: United States, 1985*. Hyattsville, MD: National Center for Health Statistics.

Institute of Medicine. (1986). *Improving the quality of care in nursing homes*. Washington, DC: National Academy Press.

Karioth, S. (1997). A loving good-bye. *Nursing Assistant Monthly, 4*(2), 2.

Kayser-Jones, J. S. (1990). *Old, alone and neglected*. Berkeley: University of California Press.

Looman, W. S., Noelker, L. S., Schur, D., Whitlatch, C. J., & Ejaz, F. K. (1997). Nursing assistants caring for dementia residents in nursing homes: The family's perspective on the high quality of care. *American Journal of Alzheimer's Disease*, 221–226.

Pillemer, K., & Moore, D. W. (1989). Abuse of patients in nursing homes: Findings from a survey of staff. *The Gerontologist, 29*(3), 314–320.

Schur, D., Noelker, L. S., Looman, W. J., Whitlatch C. J., & Ejaz, F. A (1998). Four Steps to More Committed Nursing Assistants. *American College of Health Care Administrators Balance, Jan./Feb.*, 29–31.

Strahan, G. (1987). Nursing home characteristics: Preliminary data from the 1985 Nursing Home Survey. Advance Data from Vital and Health Statistics, No. 131, Hyattsville, MD: National Center for Health Statistics.

Tellis-Nayak, V., & Tellis-Nayak, M. (1989). Quality of care and the burden of two cultures: When the world of nursing assistants enters the world of nursing homes. *The Gerontologist, 29*(3), 307–313.

Waxman, H. M., Carner, E. A., & Berkenstock, G. (1984). Job turnover and job satisfaction among nursing home aides. *The Gerontologist, 24*, 503–509.

Wilson, S. A., & Daley, B. J. (1998). Attachment/detachment: Forces influencing care of the dying in long-term care. *Journal of Palliative Medicine, 1*(1), 21–34.

3

Respect for Autonomy and the CNA

For a number of years now, respect for autonomy has been viewed as the foundation of biomedical ethics in the United States. In fact, American citizens so value this ethical principle that in 1991 respect for autonomy was institutionalized in the form of federal legislation. This legislation, the Patient Self Determination Act (PSDA), mandates that all health care facilities and home care programs that receive federal funding inform their patients or clients of their right to make treatment decisions. Particularly noteworthy is that included among these decisions is the right to refuse even life-sustaining treatment. This legislation also encourages people to execute advance directives. Such directives, generally referred to as a durable power of attorney for health care, health care proxy, or living will, either name a person to make health care decisions or outline a person's treatment preferences in the event he or she loses the ability to make decisions in the future. While many erroneously believe that the primary purpose of advance directives is to limit treatment, in reality these directives are value-neutral. Thus, through an advance directive, individuals may either opt FOR or AGAINST life-sustaining treatment.

While in theory respect for autonomy may be the dominant principle guiding health care ethics in the United States, in practice this is often not the case. Rather, anecdotal evidence suggests that paternalism often prevails in health care. Periodically, we see reports in the lay press as well as in scholarly journals suggesting that health care providers do not respect advance directives (e.g., Danis et al., 1991), the mechanism through which many attempt to exercise autonomy. Some have questioned the extent to which patients even want to exercise autonomy (e.g., High, 1988). Additionally, our work with certified nursing assistants suggests they are frequently uncomfortable with the application of the principle of autonomy. And, while to some degree this may be a function of the attitudes of the professionals with whom they work, much of this discomfort may be associated with CNAs' respective cultural backgrounds.

This chapter will address the issue of autonomy, its history in health care, and particularly how the practice of respect for autonomy may be influenced by culture. This last issue may likely be the greatest factor in determining how autonomy is viewed by CNAs, especially those drawn from a variety of countries and currently employed in nursing homes in large urban areas.

WHAT IS AUTONOMY?

As Childress (1989) reminds us, "Autonomy . . . means that a person chooses and acts freely and rationally out of her own life plan, however ill-defined" (p. 234). Inherent in this concept, he further states, are two essential elements: the ability to act freely, and the ability to deliberate rationally. Derived from the Greek *autos* (meaning "self") and *nomos* (meaning "rule" or "governance" or "law"), the term "autonomy" has been used since early Greek times. "Autonomy" has meant "a set of diverse notions including self-governance, liberty rights, privacy, individual choice, liberty to follow one's will, causing one's own behavior, and being one's own person" (Beauchamp & Childress, 1989, pp. 67–68).

Metaphorically speaking, Beauchamp and Childress (1989) tell us that an "autonomous person acts in accordance with a freely self-chosen and informed plan, just as a truly independent government acts to control its territory" (p. 68). They contrast a person of diminished autonomy with the autonomous person in that the former is, to a degree, controlled by others, or not able to deliberate or act on his or her plans. Examples of persons of diminished autonomy include prisoners, who have a severely restricted social environment, and the mentally retarded, who are limited by their psychological incapacitation. Beauchamp and Childress (1989) emphasize that while some ethicists focus on autonomous persons, it may be more useful to consider "autonomous choices." This construct of "autonomous choices" is likely a more appropriate lens through which to view the issues associated with patient care that we address with CNAs.

HISTORICAL PERSPECTIVES ON AUTONOMY

The history of ethics in health care illustrates that, for many decades, paternalism was the dominant principle. Health care providers sought to protect their patients. Thus, issues such as truth-telling, for example, were not considered, if telling the truth was thought to harm the patient. While health care providers always aimed to do good—that is, to practice the principle of beneficence, Pellegrino (1992b) reminds us that respect for autonomy has only become so dominant in the past few decades. Prior to that, he tells us, medical authoritarianism was taken for granted.

The nurse-ethicist Catherine Murphy describes changes in the nursing profession that are illustrative of the swing from medical authoritarianism to respect for autonomy in her work, "The Changing Role of Nurses in Making Ethical Decisions" (1984). Murphy discusses studies she conducted on the moral reasoning of nurses in the 1970s. At that time—only two decades ago—Murphy found the majority of nurses extremely loyal to physicians and hospitals. Only a relatively small proportion of nurses saw themselves as patient and family advocates. Over time, however, things changed markedly, with changes in society and in health care resulting in significant changes in the health care system in general and the nursing profession in particular.

Evidence of swings from paternalism toward autonomy are evident in some other countries as well, although not to the extent the pendulum has swung in the United States. For example, Surbone (1992) tells us that in the late 1970s, physicians in Italy were taught that "a serious but lethal prognosis can be hidden from the patient but not from the family" (p. 1661). By 1989, this was amended to "the physician has the duty to provide the patient—according to his cultural level and abilities to understand—the most serene information about the diagnosis, the prognosis, and the therapeutic perspectives and their consequences . . . " (p. 1661). Clearly this is a step toward autonomy. Although some may argue that many U.S. physicians still are reluctant to reveal bad news, it appears that an Italian physician's conversation with a patient newly diagnosed with a terminal illness could theoretically differ significantly from a conversation held between an American physician and a terminally ill patient.

While recognizing the value of respect for autonomy, we also need to be cautious about imposing this principle across the board. As Pellegrino (1992b) warns, in the United States autonomy has tended to become a moral absolute. This has occurred primarily as a result of improved public education, the traditional emphasis on privacy rights and personal liberty, and a distrust of authority. All of this has taken place in the context of advances in medical technology, as well as a reduction in the extent to which individuals identify themselves as members of a family or of a community. Pellegrino reminds us that respect for autonomy, as well as its corollary, truth-telling, are key features of beneficent medical care in this country.

Pellegrino (1992a) exhorts us to remember that although we ostensibly believe so strongly in respect for autonomy, we cannot assume that "this concept of autonomy . . . must always be accepted by everyone living in the United States or elsewhere" (p. 191). Rather, he suggests, those of us in health care professions must find mechanisms through which to empower patients to make decisions that reflect their values. We must let the patient decide the extent to which he or she wishes to exercise autonomy. The individual views of the patient must always be taken into consideration.

SOCIOECONOMIC ISSUES AND AUTONOMY

Where CNAs are concerned, issues associated with economics also may affect how they feel about respect for autonomy. Many CNAs are drawn from backgrounds where their socioeconomic status restricts many of the options they might have in life. In those cases, the right of people to make decisions about anything, let alone health care, have always been limited. This factor may not only make the concept of respect for autonomy difficult for CNAs to comprehend, it may set up barriers between them and those from socioeconomic groups with different life experiences who occupy our country's nursing home beds.

THE ROLE OF CULTURE AND ATTITUDES TOWARD AUTONOMY

Cultural diversity is prevalent in most American nursing homes, especially those in or near the large cities to which immigrants are traditionally drawn. This diversity is most evident in the nursing home workforce, particularly its paraprofessional component. The existence of these diverse cultures impacts not only relationships between residents and staff in nursing homes but also facilities' everyday functioning. Sensitivity to this is key to both resident satisfaction and the job satisfaction of staff in our long term care facilities.

Exploring some of the literature on culture in health care gives a sense of the magnitude of these issues. For example, in her fascinating article on cross-cultural medicine, Klessig (1992) reminds us that "many patients have immigrated from countries where as much as three-fourths of the population does not have access to basic health needs, such as clean drinking water. They have never before faced 'high-tech' health care and do not have a clear concept of the implications or consequences of initiating life support. (As well), the concept of patient autonomy that is so highly valued in Western culture, and is the basis of many life-support decisions, is not as important in other cultures" (p. 321). This description of patients from diverse cultural backgrounds also fits many certified nursing assistants, particularly those in large urban areas of the United States. Klessig and many others have examined the views of members of numerous cultures on a variety of health care issues. Their findings are relevant and can likely be generalized to health care workers from those respective cultural backgrounds.

Patients and health care providers from different cultures may hold different beliefs about health and health-related topics (Tripp-Reimer & Affifi, 1989). We find, for example, that people from different cultures describe pain differently (Morse & Morse, 1988) and present symptoms differently (Zola, 1966). Numerous studies have found patients' attitudes and choices about issues such as truth-telling, life-sustaining treatment, and euthanasia to be influenced by social and cultural values (e.g., Caralis, Davis, Wright, & Marcial, 1993). As evidenced by the work of Surbone (1992) and Blackhall, Murphy, Frank, Michel, and Azen (1995), individuals from different cultures have differing views on telling patients about terminal diagnoses. In looking at treatment decision-making for those who were unable to make decisions for themselves, members of a number of different ethnic and cultural groups felt that doctors should not make unilateral treatment decisions. Rather, decisions should always be made in concert with the family (Caralis et al., 1993).

Morrison and his colleagues (1998), using focus groups with African Americans, Hispanics, and non-Hispanic whites, found some similarities among the groups around an issue associated with autonomy: the completion of a health care proxy form. Members of all three groups exhibited a general lack of knowledge about health care proxies, and discomfort with the topic of choosing someone to make decisions when a person himself became unable to do so.

A number of researchers have looked at attitudes of specific cultural groups. While the majority of the work has been done with African Americans, we should be reminded that all African Americans cannot be lumped together, since they have varied histories. As well, recent immigrants from Africa have very different backgrounds from those whose families have resided here for longer periods of time (Klessig, 1992).

Nonetheless, in general it is believed that African Americans are less likely to agree to the limitation of life-sustaining treatment (Klessig, 1992). A number of reasons have been suggested for this, including religiosity (Klessig, 1992) and a general mistrust of the medical community (Berger, 1998; Klessig, 1992; Krakauer, 1997). As far as religion is concerned, Klessig (1992) believes that belief in a higher being may be a factor in the feelings that African Americans have toward issues such as life support. As she reminds us, for many African Americans, "a physician's statement that the situation is hopeless may not be adequate; only God knows for sure" (p. 322).

With respect to negative attitudes toward the medical community, Krakauer (1997) points out the long-standing medical racism in this country, particularly the horrors of the Tuskegee Syphilis Study, as well as evidence that African Americans continue to be denied adequate medical services. This builds upon the fact that African Americans had been enslaved, segregated, and discriminated against. In short, their experience is illustrative of institutionalized racism. How can they logically expect fairness and consideration in the health care system? As Berger (1998) reminds us, in contrast to the white majority, who worry about receiving too much treatment at the end of life, many African Americans have concerns about undertreatment. Even discussion of issues associated with end of life decision-making is perceived negatively by many African Americans. This is particularly unfortunate, since African Americans are more likely than the general population to suffer from conditions such as cancer and cardiovascular diseases where such discussions could be very useful (Klessig, 1992).

Often, members of socially vulnerable groups have difficulty with issues related to medical care and autonomy. Morrow (1997), in studying some of these individuals (older persons, Latinas who do not speak English, homeless women, and women who were victims of domestic violence), found members of these groups to be extremely suspicious of the medical community. Specifically, they expressed concern about physicians' desire to increase their incomes, they felt that many doctors are corrupt, and that they treat indigent people very differently from their economically-comfortable counterparts.

In looking at groups of individuals representing a number of other cultures, major differences were found between them and the majority culture in the United States on a number of issues related to health care and often to autonomy. For example, Carrese and Rhodes (1995), in studying Navaho Indians, found that 86 percent of their subjects believed that advance care planning was a violation of Navaho values. Clearly, caution should be exercised by health care providers attempting to discuss these issues with Navahos who will understandably resist executing advance directives or even discussing future treatment preferences. Concrete manifestation of respect for autonomy through the use of advance directives is something alien to members of other cultures. As Berger (1998) reminds us, "Implicit in a dependency on the use of advance directives for health decisions are the assumptions that a future orientation toward life and health is universal, and that individualism is of uniform importance. However, many minorities embrace an orientation toward life that focuses more on the present moment" (p. 127).

Klessig (1992), commenting on Iranians, notes that the concept of options and patient autonomy is unknown in traditional Iranian culture. Since Iranian patients are not accustomed to making choices, they may delay doing so. In the Iranian culture, the physician makes the decision. Therefore, in the health care setting, asking an Iranian patient to make decisions about treatment may be a frustrating experience for both the patient and the health care provider.

Klessig's (1992) work with Koreans suggests that they perceive stopping life support as interfering with God's will. Traditional attitudes toward longevity may discourage Koreans from limiting life-sustaining treatment. Older people in Korea are held in such high esteem that Korea has a national "Respect for the Elderly" Week (Sung, 1990). The Korean belief in filial piety mandates that children's responsibility toward parents is paramount, and asking that life support be discontinued is viewed as wrong.

Many Chinese, it has been suggested, believe that near the end of life, nature (in the form of death) should be allowed to take its course, and Chinese have traditionally found it acceptable to choose death (Klessig, 1992). Additionally, in Chinese culture, every individual is viewed as a part of a greater whole. Therefore, consideration must be given to the effect of an individual's illness on the family. Accordingly, financial issues associated with treating end-stage illness come into play in the decision-making process. It is believed that

Buddha emphasized justice and compassion. A patient's decision to forgo life support may prevent his family from financial and emotional suffering. This, then, is good.

Clearly, a knowledge of the impact of cultural values is key in the health care setting. This holds true not only for the patient, but also for the health care provider, both professional and paraprofessional. In the United States, we must be aware that we care for patients from a variety of cultural backgrounds, and we are cared for by health care providers from a variety of cultural backgrounds. Knowledge of these differences, and how they play out with respect to ethical principles, is key. As Surbone (1992) reminds us, beneficence in one country may be maleficence in another.

We need to be aware that with health care, conflicts may arise between patient and provider. Knowledge that mistrust related to social inequalities, racism and cultural differences may interfere with the therapeutic relationship is the first step to improving that relationship (Krakauer, 1997).

Randall (1994), writing on ethnic Americans and the Patient Self Determination Act, cautions us that the PSDA promotes individual autonomy. Some may view this as its greatest benefit, while others may see it as a major liability. Respect for autonomy may be the norm in the mainstream United States (assuming there is such a thing as a mainstream United States). Nonetheless, it is in conflict with the traditional family decision-making that is inherent in most cultures. We should take care not to forget that in fact, family decision-making was the norm historically in the United States as well. The PSDA is often quite ineffective for persons who are not European-American, middle-class, and middle-aged. Thus, Randall (1994) suggests that, when attempting to implement the PSDA with Americans drawn from other cultures, a number of issues must be considered. These include awareness of communication and language barriers, attitudes toward death and dying, and attitudes about the body. Religious beliefs about the meaningfulness of suffering also come into play, as does the family's role in decision making and the trust (or lack of it) in the health care system.

In fact, attitudes toward family decision-making are deeply ingrained in many cultures, as well as in members of vulnerable groups. Morrow (1997), for example, found individuals both from minority cultures and disadvantaged backgrounds believing strongly in the family. They stressed that families would act in their best interests, and that they should always be involved in health care decisions. In fact, families could act as a check on the power of physicians, who could not always be trusted. While many of Morrow's subjects felt the right to make choices was important, choices related to end-of-life care should be made within the context of the family.

Berger (1998) notes in writing about health care decision-making in New York State that the model of patient care that is based on respect for autonomy excludes "models in which intra-family fealty and physicians' fiduciary responsibilities are valued" (p. 129). Unfortunately, all too often the cultural majority is favored in the manner by which we make medical decisions and the processes by which treatments are limited. This can have a profound impact upon the patient population. It may also cause philosophical difficulties for health care providers from other countries and other cultures.

Klessig (1992) makes a number of suggestions for those in health care to consider when dealing with individuals from different cultural backgrounds. These recommendations are particularly relevant when making health care decisions in a setting where autonomous choice is considered the norm. Specifically, Klessig reminds us to try to determine how the individual feels about the sanctity of life. How do they define death? What are their religious beliefs, if any? And how religious are they? What do they think caused their illness, and is this related to the dying process? What about their social support system, and who makes decisions of importance where they or their family members are concerned?

WHAT DOES ALL THIS MEAN FOR THE CERTIFIED NURSING ASSISTANT?

What is most evident when thinking about CNAs and our current perspectives on autonomy is that many CNAs find acceptance of this concept troublesome, either for themselves or for the residents to whom they render care and with whom they develop close emotional attachments. When manifestations of autonomy are closely intertwined with limiting life-sustaining treatment, CNAs may be particularly troubled. The thought that an individual may choose not to receive treatment that may keep him or her alive is incomprehensible to many CNAs for a variety of reasons.

One may be the influence of other health care personnel. In our work with the Ethics Consult Team at The Jewish Home and Hospital (Chichin & Olson, 1995; Olson, Chichin, Meyers, Schulman, & Brennan, 1994), we regularly encountered nurses, often from other cultures, who clearly have difficulty when residents opt to limit life-sustaining treatment. The often unspoken sentiment is that life-sustaining technology must be used. In fact, techniques such as artificial nutrition and hydration are seen as the norm by many nurses. Additionally, many anecdotal experiences with physicians in hospitals mirror this viewpoint. Opinions of the professionals with whom they associate may clearly influence the thinking of CNAs.

What is particularly striking about this phenomenon is that when CNAs from other countries were asked what would be done in their own country, they tell us that feeding tubes are not used in their countries. Nor, as a matter of fact, are nursing homes. Rather, families keep their old people at home with them. Statements to this effect were made repeatedly in a study of staff feelings about treatment termination in nursing homes (Chichin & Olson, 1998). For example:

> I come from Jamaica and when you have your family there and they're old we don't use nursing homes. Everybody's family takes care of who they have at home. They want to be at home.

> (I'm from the West Indies and) when I was there they didn't have any (nursing homes). Most of the elderly were kept at home. There is always someone to take care of them.

> Well honestly, in the Dominican Republic we don't really believe in nursing homes. We believe in taking care of our own. They can even go senile and we take care of them at home. That's the way it is over there. I had a grandmother who was senile and we kept her at home also. (Here, it is different). In the beginning, I thought it was just that people were abandoning their families and it bothered me a lot. But after a while I learned to accept that some people just can't handle it. Especially here we live in a whole different society. Here everything is a rush. You barely have time for yourself, let alone taking care of someone who needs a lot of care.

Clearly, the influence of one's respective culture plays a prominent role in how one views autonomy. As noted earlier, different cultures place different emphases on various ethical principles, and the thinking on these issues in the mainstream United States does not generally reflect thinking world-wide.

Yet another issue may simply be the way we typically interpret the meaning of the term autonomy. Surbone (1992) notes that clinicians in a number of cultures are treating patients who are quite aware of the gravity of their conditions. Discussing this, however, is not an acceptable practice, and patients make a choice not to engage in such conversations. The fact that this choice is made, Surbone reminds us, is one way of exercising autonomy.

In conclusion, while autonomy may be the dominant principle in American biomedical ethics, there are numerous factors involved in how CNAs feel about this concept, and how it impacts upon them personally and in their work lives. As Rempusheski (1989) reminds us, "There are Western scientific beliefs, and individuals' ethnic and religious beliefs, and ethical beliefs underlying (one's) profession" (p. 722). Together or separately, each of these may influence how CNAs view respect for autonomy.

While we can teach CNAs about the concept of respect for autonomy, there are numerous barriers to their ability to accept and apply this ethical principle, both for themselves and for those they care for. Issues associated with autonomy are many, and in the nursing home setting, far exceed issues limited to withholding and withdrawing life-sustaining treatment. In discussing the concept of autonomy with CNAs, it is important to mention not only issues around advance directives, but also the everyday issues that come up in routine care of nursing home residents. What they wear, where they sit in the dining room, what activities they attend, all are part of their exercise of autonomy. CNAs assume responsibility for the majority of hands-on care of residents who may be dying because they have opted to not receive a feeding tube. They also, however, have control over myriad everyday aspects of a resident's life. This is an issue that should be emphasized to CNAs.

REFERENCES

Beauchamp, T. L., & Childress, J. F. (1989). *Principles of biomedical ethics* (3rd ed.). New York: Oxford University Press.

Berger, J. T. (1998). Cultural discrimination in mechanisms for health decisions: A view from New York. *Journal of Clinical Ethics, 9*(2), 127–131.

Blackhall, L. J., Murphy, S. T., Frank, G., Michel, V., & Azen, S. (1995). Ethnicity and attitudes toward patient autonomy. *Journal of the American Medical Association, 274*(10), 820–825.

Caralis, P. V., Davis, B., Wright, K., & Marcial, E. (1993). The influence of race and ethnicity on attitudes toward advance directives, life-prolonging treatment and euthanasia. *Journal of Clinical Ethics, 4*(2), 155–165.

Carrese, J. A., & Rhodes, L. A. (1995). Western bioethics on the Navajo reservation: Benefit or harm? *Journal of the American Medical Association, 274*(10), 826–829.

Chichin, E. R., & Olson, E. (1995). An ethics consult team in geriatric long-term care. *Cambridge Quarterly of Healthcare Ethics* (4), 178–184.

Chichin, E. R., & Olson, E. (1998). Staff reactions to dementia patients' requests to withhold or withdraw treatment. *Final Report to the New York State Department of Health Bureau of Long-term Care Dementia Grants Project.*

Childress, J. (1989). Autonomy. In R. M. Veatch (Ed.), *Cross-cultural perspectives in medical ethics: Readings* (pp. 233–241). Boston: Jones and Bartlett.

Danis, M., Southerland, L. I., Garrett, J. M., Smith, J. L., Hielema, F., Pickard, C. G., Egner, D. M., & Patrick, D. L. (1991). A prospective study of advance directives for life-sustaining care. *New England Journal of Medicine, 324*(13), 882–888.

High, D. (1988). All in the family: Extended autonomy and expectations in surrogate health care decision-making. *Gerontologist, 28*(Suppl.), 46–51.

Klessig, J. (1992). Cross-cultural medicine a decade later. *Western Journal of Medicine, 157*, 316–322.

Krakauer, E. L. (1997). Commentary. *Hastings Center Report (May-June)*, 23–24.

Morrison, R. S., Zayas, L. H., Mulvihill, M., Baskin, S., & Meier, D. E. (1998). Barriers to completion of health care proxy forms: A qualitative analysis of ethnic differences. *Journal of Clinical Ethics, 9*(2), 118–126.

Morrow, E. (1997). Attitudes of women from vulnerable populations to physician-assisted suicide: A qualitative approach. *Journal of Clinical Ethics, 8*(3), 279–289.

Morse, J. M., & Morse, R. M. (1988). Cultural variation in the inference of pain. *Journal of Cross-cultural Psychology, 19*(2), 232–242.

Murphy, C. (1984). The changing role of nurses in making ethical decisions. *Law, Medicine, and Health Care, 12*, 173–174, 184.

Olson, E., Chichin, E. R., Meyers, H., Schulman, E., & Brennan, F. (1994). Early experiences of an ethics consult team. *Journal of the American Geriatrics Society, 42*, 437–441.

Pellegrino, E. D. (1992a). Intersections of western biomedical ethics and world culture: Problematic and possibility. *Cambridge Quarterly of Healthcare Ethics* (3), 191–196.

Pellegrino, E. D. (1992b). Is truth-telling to the patient a cultural artifact? *Journal of the American Medical Association, 268*(13), 1734–1735.

Randall, V. R. (1994). Ethnic Americans, long-term health care providers, and the Patient Self Determination Act. In M. B. Kapp (Ed.), *Patient Self-Determination in Long-term Care* (pp. 123–141). New York: Springer.

Rempusheski, V. F. (1989). The role of ethnicity in elder care. *Nursing Clinics of North America, 24*(3), 717–724.

Sung, K. (1990). A new look at filial piety: Ideals and practices of family-centered patient care in Korea. *Gerontologist, 30*(5), 610–617.

Surbone, A. (1992). Letter from Italy: Truth telling to the patient. *Journal of the American Medical Association, 268*(13), 1661–1662.

Tripp-Reimer, T., & Afifi, L. A. (1989). Cross-cultural perspectives in patient teaching. *Nursing Clinics of North America, 24*(3), 613–619.

Zola, I. K. (1966). Culture and symptoms: An analysis of patients presenting complaints. *American Sociological Review, 31*(5), 615–630.

4

Comfort Care

INTRODUCTION

In working with the CNAs involved in this project, we used the term "comfort care" when discussing how to provide appropriate care to the dying. Our intention in focusing on comfort care was to communicate to them basic principles of palliative care, drawing both on what has been published to date on this vital topic, as well as our own experience in care of the dying in the long term care setting (Chichin & Olson, 1997). This chapter is an overview of some of the key concepts of palliative care, many of which were included in the educational program for the CNAs in this project.For purposes of this chapter, the terms "comfort care" and "palliative care" will be used interchangeably.

To place the concept of palliative care in historical context, this is a term that essentially came into vogue in the late 1980s when, in Great Britain, palliative medicine became a specialty practiced by physicians. It has been recognized, however, that palliative care is best provided by an interdisciplinary team consisting of a number of professionals, paraprofessionals, and volunteers (Doyle, Hanks, & MacDonald, 1994). As described by the World Health Organization (1990), palliative care is defined as:

> "The active total care of patients whose disease is not responsive to curative treatment. Control of pain, of other symptoms, and the psychological, social and spiritual problems, is paramount. The goal of palliative care is achievement of the best quality of life for patients and their families."

Doyle et al. (1994), in their superb volume, *Oxford Textbook of Palliative Medicine*, remind us that the concept of palliative care clearly was an offspring of hospice care. "Hospice care," however, implies care of the terminally ill, and there are many issues around the ability to clearly define the word "terminal." Accordingly, Doyle and his colleagues utilized the term "palliative medicine" rather than "hospice" or "terminal care" when writing this important volume. As they so eloquently state, " 'Terminal' care suggests a preoccupation with dying and death, grief, loss, and sadness and, although we do not wish to create a sanitizing definition, the care outlined in (the *Oxford Textbook of Palliative Medicine*) affirms life rather than death" (Doyle et al., 1994, p. 3).

It is this thinking, in part, that we wished to communicate to the certified nursing assistants participating in this project. Additionally, we wished to disabuse them of myths associated with care of the dying (e.g., that artificial nutrition and hydration are comfort measures), and educate them about the key role that CNAs play in providing palliative care to nursing home residents. As well, we sought to raise their awareness of the fact that palliative care principles can appropriately be applied throughout a resident's nursing home stay, not only during the dying process.

BACKGROUND

Certified nursing assistants, like their professional counterparts, tend to be enamored of medical technology. As a rule, they perceive the use of intravenous therapies and tube feedings as taking precedence over such non-technical tasks such as bathing, toileting, and feeding by mouth. The provision of emotional support, through such things as talking to the resident and hand-holding, is relegated to a relatively low position in the caregiving hierarchy. Thus, there is a tendency to minimize a great deal of what CNAs do with respect to patient or resident care. As Slomka (1995) reminds us, we have come to equate care of the patient with medical care of the patient. Disabusing CNAs, as well as physicians and nurses, of the fact that only high-tech medical care has any value is a challenge not easily met.

Fortunately, there is a movement afoot across the United States to humanize care of both the living and the dying through the application of palliative care principles. Indications of increased attention to applying the principles of palliative care are numerous, and include Dr. Joanne Lynn's *Americans for Better Care of the Dying* (ABCD), as well as financier George Soros' *Project on Death in America* as two notable examples. Unfortunately, however, when one enters the "trenches" where the majority of health care is being provided (hospitals and nursing homes) there is difficulty in changing the mind-set that prioritizes more technical aspects of care. The more we are able to raise the awareness of the public in general and health care providers in particular about the use of palliative care and to apply its principles in appropriate situations, the more we will be able to humanize the dying process. Accordingly, one of the goals of this project was to educate CNAs about comfort care while emphasizing the key role that they play in providing it.

NURSING HOME RESIDENTS AND THE DYING PROCESS

In his useful volume on medical care of the terminally ill, Enck (1994) described the terminal process as " . . . a continuous process as the body and brain are unable to cope with hypoxia, malnutrition, electrolyte imbalance, tumor burden (in the case of cancer), and toxins that are not cleared from the body as hepatic and renal failure occur. Emotion, cognition, thinking, behavior, and autonomic function all slowly deteriorate and, in most cases, coma ensues before death" (p. 161). Enck also tells us that, while studies suggest that about one-third of dying patients appear to experience some discomfort in their final days, this can usually be adequately managed by reassurance or pharmacological therapies.

The deaths of nursing home residents may result from a number of causes, including major cardiovascular conditions, malignant neoplasms, infectious diseases, pneumonia and other conditions (U.S. Department of Health and Human Services, 1992). While a major goal of nursing home care should be to maintain the resident or patient at the highest level of comfort possible, this is an even greater priority when someone is dying. It has been suggested that no matter what the underlying illness, when patients are very close to death (i.e., during the last 48 to 72 hours of life), about one-third to one-half experience disturbing symptoms. Among these are noisy, moist breathing and pain, as well as agitation and restlessness (Enck, 1994). Mechanisms to address these symptoms are generally readily available in the health care setting, and should be utilized appropriately whenever necessary. Unfortunately, they are used all too infrequently.

In addition to the conditions mentioned above as causes of death of nursing home patients, a significant majority suffer from Alzheimer's disease or other dementing illnesses. Care of the nursing home patient can be difficult at best; when compounded by dementia it is even more complex. When a dementing illness reaches its end stages, care of the patient is an even greater challenge, since the final phases of these conditions render their victims unable to speak (Reisberg, Ferris, DeLeon, & Crook, 1982). Thus, patients with dementing illnesses are unable to complain of discomfort. As a result, the existence of pain can only be inferred. Of concern here is that these patients' inability to communicate pain or discomfort may result in the failure of their health care providers to intervene when patients are suffering distressing problems. In the worst case scenario, health care providers in long term care may perceive individuals dying from terminal dementia as neonates once were viewed: unable to feel pain (Purcell Jones, Dormon, & Sumner, 1987; 1988; Truog & Hickey, 1991).

There is reason to assume that patients dying from end-stage dementias, like those dying from the conditions mentioned earlier, will experience similar symptoms at the end of life. Since they cannot verbalize their discomfort, health care providers must be particularly sensitive to nuances that may indicate distress. While breathing patterns, restlessness and agitation are obvious to the observer (and may, in fact, be an indication of pain), in general the assessment of pain in patients with impaired communication is a particularly difficult challenge (AHCPR, 1992a; APS, 1992; McCaffrey, 1993). As Hodges and Tolle (1994) remind us, "severe pain may be communicated through grimaces, crying, moaning, and other body language, but the gestures and the expressions can be difficult to interpret" (p. 481). Querying those who know the patient best—his or her family or care givers— regarding the patient's level of discomfort may be helpful in coming to some determination of whether the patient has pain (Enck, 1994; McCaffrey, 1993). While we may never be sure if an uncommunicative patient is experiencing pain, anecdotal reports suggest that many compassionate clinicians prefer to err on the side of keeping the patient comfortable and readily use analgesics.

THE USE OF COMFORT CARE

As Field and Cassel (1997) remind us, there are four dimensions of care at the end of life: the physical, the emotional, the spiritual, and the practical. With respect to the physical, comfort is clearly an overriding issue. Thus, we must attend to symptom management, as well as hygiene, nutritional status, and maintenance of skin integrity. Under the psychological dimension, issues of both cognitive function and emotional status come into play. The spiritual dimension often involves "a search for meaning, peace, or transcendence that can replace fear and despair with hope and serenity" (Field & Cassel, 1997, p. 78). And finally, in looking at the practical dimension of care of the dying, which often overlaps with the physical, the emotional, and the spiritual, this includes issues such as knowledge of the condition and treatment, issues around decision-making, and who to contact to manage the myriad issues associated with care of the dying, including what to do after death. Also included in the practical dimension are issues associated with the physical environment and personal care, concerns about the burdens of caregiving borne by the family, financial and other practical issues such as household maintenance.

BASIC COMPONENTS OF COMFORT CARE

Educating CNAs about their roles in the delivery of palliative care should begin with a user-friendly overview of the major components of palliative care. Given the interdisciplinary nature of palliative care, as well as the discipline-specific or educational limitations placed on different individuals involved in its provision, CNAs, although key players, will clearly not be directly involved in all aspects of palliative care. For example, CNAs will not be administering medication. Nonetheless, they should be aware of the use of a variety of medications for pain control, as well as their role in observing a resident's response to attempts to control pain. Accordingly, this chapter will present an overview of some key aspects of palliative care, including pain and symptom control, as well as emotional and spiritual needs associated with appropriate care of the dying.

Pain and Symptom Management

Assessment of Pain

An issue of great concern, and one that is often overlooked or minimized in health care in general, is appropriate pain control. In one disturbing report, nurses stated that they felt the most serious form of drug abuse in hospitals was the undertreatment of pain (Solomon et al., 1993). Fortunately, we are seeing increased attention to the awareness of pain. Of note is the new trend in health care institutions of including pain as "the fifth vital sign" (i.e., after blood pressure, temperature, pulse and respirations, the existence of pain will be assessed).

In patients in general and particularly in terminally ill patients, adequate pain management is imperative (Enck, 1994). Appropriate management of pain is a challenge in many situations, and practitioners may find it useful to follow guidelines developed by the American Pain Society (1995). Included among their recommendations are the following:

1. the recognition and prompt treatment of pain
2. maintaining a patient's self-report of pain initially and after each intervention used to relieve pain
3. documentation of patient's perceptions of care
4. provision of process and outcomes of pain management to the health care team
5. sharing of information about pain control and analgesics with all health care providers

6. developing educational programs, competencies, monitoring techniques, and policies for the use of more advanced pain-relieving technologies (such as patient controlled infusions)
7. utilize continuous quality improvement techniques to assess pain management

While these suggestions are extremely useful in all health care settings, they present unique challenges in care of the elderly and especially in care of the elderly dying in nursing homes. This population, while somewhat varied with respect to diagnostic category, suffers from a number of conditions clearly associated with the existence of pain. Complicating this situation to an even greater degree, as mentioned above, is the high proportion of this population affected by dementing illness. Among those suffering from Alzheimer's disease or related disorders, the ability to communicate discomfort wanes as the disease progresses. Therefore, a heightened awareness of any manifestation of discomfort is key.

Pain Management

A commonly-used approach to the management of pain in patients with cancer diagnoses has been recommended by the World Health Organization (WHO) (Enck, 1994; Doyle et al., 1994). This "ladder" approach is also useful in care of those dying from other conditions. The WHO ladder begins with non-opiod drugs such as acetaminophen (Tylenol) and non-steroidal anti-inflammatory preparations (NSAIDS) such as aspirin, ibuprofen, fenoprofen, and naproxen. These medications are appropriate for mild to moderate pain, and are used orally (with the exception of acetaminophen and aspirin, which can also be administered via rectal suppository). The advantage of these drugs is that repeated administration is not associated with tolerance and physical dependence. However, additional pain control will not occur with increased doses beyond a certain level (Enck, 1994), and these drugs also may have side effects.

If pain should persist, a move up the ladder to a weak opiod such as codeine or oxycodone is recommended. If pain continues to be a problem, a stronger opiod, such as morphine, is indicated. In all cases of severe pain, a strong opiod should be used. When needed, especially in cancer pain, adjuvant analgesics may also be used. Adjuvant analgesics include preparations such as anticonvulsants, phenothiazines, and tricyclic antidepressants. The mechanism by which they relieve pain is generally not understood (Enck, 1994).

A key issue in appropriate pain control is to avoid "p.r.n" or "as needed" dosing. The administration of pain medication when pain occurs (in contrast to round-the-clock dosing) results in uneven analgesia, which is referred to as a "peak and trough" effect on blood levels. Administering analgesics around the clock, starting with the lowest possible dose and titrating upward as needed, provides a constant level of comfort (Enck, 1994). Oral administration is preferred whenever possible, and combinations of drugs often are more effective than a single drug.

Another important issue is the awareness of side effects. A most commonly seen condition in nursing home residents is constipation; this becomes an even greater concern with the use of opiods. Therefore, appropriate bowel regimens should be initiated when opiods are used. As well, given the high use of medications with anticholinergic side effects in this population, dry mouth is another common occurrence, and frequent mouth care is strongly recommended.

Other Symptoms

The other most frequently-occurring symptoms, particularly in the last few days of life, are tachypnea (rapid breathing) and possibly restlessness. Observing a resident with very rapid breathing is often very distressing to family members and to staff. The most effective drug for tachypnea is morphine, which may be used intravenously, subcutaneously, orally, or via G-tube. For chronic tachypnea, a transdermal opiod (i.e., fentanyl) can be used. As is the rule with a frail elderly population, the smallest possible dose should be initiated (generally 2 to 4 milligrams subcutaneously, or its equivalent), but this can be increased as needed. Some clinicians use respiratory parameters, administering morphine for respirations faster that 25 per minute, and holding the dose for a rate less than 10 or 12.

Morphine is also useful for restlessness, particularly if it is assumed that pain may be the cause. However, Ativan (lorazepam) is frequently also effective.

Dry mouth, mentioned above as a side effect of anticholiniergic medications, is almost always present in the dying. As mentioned frequently in this volume, the work of McCann and his colleagues (1994) with dying cancer patients who were able to communicate their discomfort is particularly noteworthy. Most significant were their complaints of dry mouth, and the fact that this can be relieved with meticulous mouth care, ice chips, and small sips of water as tolerated. This is an issue that must be emphasized with CNAs. Assuming that pain is controlled, the symptom that may be most distressing to dying patients is dry mouth. This is a symptom readily addressed by nursing assistants who provide most of the hands-on care and who are generally directly responsible for this aspect of care.

Skin breakdown, a key issue in nursing homes, may also occur near death, especially with older people who are poorly nourished. Regular positioning is an important component of care of the dying to prevent the development of bedsores which can heighten discomfort.

Emotional support is another key aspect of comprehensive care of the dying. While many of the residents who die in nursing homes suffer from advanced dementia and are unable to communicate, they nonetheless often appear to be comforted by gentle touching and hand-holding. The sound of familiar voices may also provide solace, and staff should be encouraged to continue to talk to and touch dying residents.

The provision of spiritual support may also provide comfort to dying residents, and the knowledge that clergy are in attendance certainly may help family members.

Other measures that should be considered when caring for dying residents include any other intervention that may provide comfort or a sense of peace. If the resident enjoyed music, for example, attempts should be made to have the music of choice available.

FAMILY SUPPORT

In a study of dying dementia patients conducted in 1995 and 1996 at The Jewish Home and Hospital in New York City (Chichin & Olson, 1997), perhaps the most significant finding was the profound effect of the dying process of patients on their surviving family members, as well as the caregiving staff. The concerns of a family around a resident's dying and imminent death are many. The emotional impact on families is particularly intense when the dying process is associated with a resident's previously expressed wishes for the withholding or withdrawing of artificial nutrition and hydration.

When the use of artificial nutrition and hydration (tube feedings and intravenous therapy) is limited, families often assume that death will occur in a day or two. This is rarely the case, and the dying process often lasts substantially longer. This waiting period, and watching the resident die, even in cases where there is no obvious discomfort associated with the process, is very difficult for families. Even in cases where the family is convinced that they are carrying out the resident's wishes, they question the decision to withhold or withdraw artificial nutrition. In our work with the Ethics Consult Team at The Jewish Home and Hospital, we have had the experience of families telling us they felt like executioners. And, the longer it takes for death to occur, the more distressed families become.

Families need to be reminded that the decision to limit the use of life-sustaining treatment very often is not theirs, but rather that of their relative. This is particularly the case in New York State, where treatment decisions for adults can only be made by the individual himself or herself, either at the time the decision needs to be made or in advance via a written or oral directive or the appointment of a proxy decision-maker. In other states, where families have more leeway to make treatment decisions for incapacitated relatives, these decisions are not made lightly, and are generally decided upon using best interest or benefit versus burden assessments. Thus, families should be reminded of this, and of the fact that they are acting as agents to insure either fulfilling the resident's previously expressed wishes, or, assuming they have received appropriate medical advice, what is best for the resident. Additionally, the family must be reassured that the dying resident is being kept very comfortable, and all manifestations of discomfort have been and will be addressed.

Professional and paraprofessional health care providers in nursing homes also need to address with families the myth that people dying without artificial nutrition and hydration are "starving to death." There is currently an abundance of literature that suggests strongly that withholding or withdrawing artificial nutrition and hydration results in death from dehydration, which is believed to be a most comfortable way to die (Ahronheim, 1996; Billings, 1985; Brody, Campbell, Faber-Langdon, & Ogle, 1997; McCann, Hall, & Groth-Juncker, 1994; Oliver, 1992; Printz, 1992; Zerweckh, 1983; 1987; 1997). In fact, it appears that dying in a dehydrated state is significantly more comfortable than dying artificially hydrated. Changes in the body's chemistry during the process of dehydration cause a natural sedation. Additionally, avoiding the use of artificial hydration minimizes secretions, thereby decreasing the need for suctioning, a procedure that many family members find distressing. As well, eliminating the use of intravenous therapies means the dying resident will not be subjected to repeated venipunctures.

STAFF SUPPORT

As noted above, staff distress was another one of the most significant findings of our study of the comfort level of dying dementia patients (Chichin & Olson, 1997). Vachon (1994), in writing on emotional problems in palliative medicine, noted, "Not only do patients and their families suffer distress, so too do those who care for them" (p. 579). She tells of an early study where she and her colleagues found nurses starting a palliative care unit experiencing distress as high as that of women who were newly widowed. The distress of these women was even higher than that of women with newly diagnosed breast cancer who were undergoing radiation (Lyall, Vachon, & Rogers, 1980).

The stress that staff feel may be a function of working with dying persons in general or the death of a one (or more) patient(s) in particular. Vachon (1994) believes this may come from a variety of sources: from the person himself or herself as a result of life experiences, or because of the death of a particular patient, or perhaps from "death overload"—too many patients dying in a brief period of time, as well as too great an investment in patients.

Vachon (1994) also found other factors that are related to the work environment possibly contributing to stress in caring for the dying. These include unrealistic expectations of what can be accomplished, or insufficient resources to carry out one's work. Some of the variables Vachon (1994) suggests influence the degree to which those caring for the dying experience stress include age, personality, social support, and stressful life events. With respect to age, younger workers seem to have more manifestations of stress, as well as fewer coping mechanisms. Personality characteristics that seem to mitigate the stressful effects of working with the dying include having a sense of commitment, feelings about the meaningfulness of life, having a sense of control (as opposed to feeling powerless), and believing that it is normal for life to change (Kobasa, Maddi, & Courington, 1981).

All staff who are involved with the end-stage nursing home resident are affected to some degree by the resident's dying process. In our work at The Jewish Home and Hospital, those most distressed appear to be physicians, nurses, and certified nursing assistants. However, other disciplines (therapists, dietitians, etc.) who have had close relationships with the resident may also be affected by the impending death. Therefore, their responses should also be considered when education and emotional support are being provided. Team meetings, particularly those where CNAs are in attendance, are the optimum venue for discussions of these issues.

Many of the concerns expressed by staff members caring for dying residents mirror those of families. Specifically, staff may question whether the resident is starving to death. Many voice the desire to "at least" start an IV. Staff, too, are distressed by the length of the dying process. They may also question how we can be sure that what we are doing is what the resident would have wanted. Given the regularity with which they see feeding tubes being used, they often do not perceive their use as burdensome, and may minimize the unpleasant aspects (and potential dangers) of artificial nutrition and hydration.

It may be useful to suggest to staff that they try to consider what they know of the resident as a person, and specifically what the resident's values may have been. They should then apply this information to the resident's current situation, and decide for themselves what they think the resident would have wanted. If this information is not known, for example if they had never known the resident prior to advanced dementia, they must recognize that, by law, we are obligated to respect whatever the resident expressed via oral or written advance directives.

Another issue we have encountered in our work with staff caring for dying residents, particularly when the death is associated with a dementing illness, is the reluctance of nurses (and the resultant effect on CNAs) to use narcotics. Despite the fact that the doses used for dying dementia patients with tachypnea, for example, are minuscule, nurses often express concern about "putting the patient over the edge." We have found that ongoing education and constant emotional support are useful here, with an emphasis on our responsibility to keep dying residents comfortable.

CONCLUSION

It is unfortunate that the experience of dying in this country has been medicalized to such a great degree. This, in concert with insufficient expertise in pain and symptom control and management, is most likely the primary reason why both professionals and paraprofessionals in our health care system tend to minimize the importance of many components of comfort care. While pain and symptom management are the foundation of comprehensive palliative (or comfort) care, too many health care providers fail to recognize the importance of such rudimentary acts as turning and positioning a patient, touching and hand-holding, and just talking to a patient. Additionally, as noted earlier, the use of meticulous mouth care cannot be overemphasized. These seemingly simple things can provide an immeasurable level of comfort and support to someone who is dying. Recognizing this may provide some level of solace to staff, who realize that they can replace the use of aggressive life-sustaining treatment with equally important comfort care. CNAs should be particularly consoled by the realization that their role in comfort care is one of the most vital.

REFERENCES

AHCPR. (1992a). Acute pain management in adults operative procedures. *Quick reference guide for clinicians*. Pub. No. 92-0019.

AHCPR. (1992b). Acute pain management in infants, children, and adolescents: Operative and medical procedures. *Quick reference guide for clinicians*. Pub. No. 92-0020.

Ahronheim, J. (1996). Nutrition and hydration in the terminal patient. *Clinics in Geriatric Medicine, 12*(2), 379–391.

American Pain Society (APS). (1992). *Principles of analgesic use in the treatment of acute pain and cancer pain* (3rd ed.). Skokie, IL: The Society.

American Pain Society (APS). (1995). Quality Improvement Guidelines for the Treatment of Acute Pain and Cancer Pain. *Journal of the American Medical Association, 274*, 1874–1880.

Billings, J. A. (1985). Comfort measures for the terminally ill: Is dehydration painful? *Journal of the American Geriatrics Society, 33*(11), 808–810.

Brody, H., Campbell, M. L., Faber-Langendoen, K., & Ogle, K. S. (1997). Withdrawing intensive life-sustaining treatment: Recommendations for compassionate clinical management. *New England Journal of Medicine, 366*(9), 652–657.

Chichin, E. R., & Olson, E. (1997). The dying process of end-stage dementia patients: Can we make it better? *Final Report to the New York State Department of Health Bureau of Long-term Care Services 1994 Dementia Grants Project.*

Doyle, D., Hanks, G., & MacDondald, N. (1994). Introduction. In D. Doyle, G. Hanks, & N. MacDonald (Eds.), *Oxford Textbook of Palliative Medicine* (pp. 3–8). New York: Oxford University Press.

Enck, R. E. (1994). *Medical care of the terminally ill.* Baltimore, MD: Johns Hopkins University Press.

Field, M. J., & Cassel, C. K. (1997). *Approaching death: Improving care at the end of life.* Washington, DC: National Academy Press.

Hodges, M. O., & Tolle, S. W. (1994). Tube feeding decisions in the elderly. *Clinics in Geriatric Medicine, 10*(3), 475–488.

Kobasa, S. C., Maddi, S. R., & Courington, S. (1981). Personality and constitution as mediators in the stress-illness relationship. *Journal of Health and Social Behavior, 37*, 1–11.

Lyall, A., Vachon, M., & Rogers, J. (1980). A study of the degree of stress experienced by professionals caring for dying patients. In I. Ajemian and B. M. Mount (Eds.), *The RVH Manual on Palliative/Hospice Care* (pp. 498–508). New York: ARNO Press.

McCaffrey, M. (1993). Pain: Assessment and intervention in clinical practice. Unpublished syllabus.

McCann, R. M., Hall, W. J., & Groth-Juncker, A. (1994). Comfort care for terminally ill patients: The appropriate use of nutrition and hydration. *Journal of the American Medical Association, 272*(16), 1263–1266.

Oliver, D. (1984). Terminal dehydration. *Lancet, II*(8403), 631.

Printz, L.A. (1992). Terminal dehydration: A compassionate treatment. *Archives of Internal Medicine, 152*, 697–700.

Purcell Jones, G., Dormon, F., & Sumner, E. (1987). Paediatric anaesthetists' perceptions of neonatal and infant pain. *Pain, 33*, 181–187.

Purcell Jones, G., Dormon, F., & Sumner, E. (1988). The use of opioids in neonates: A retrospective study of 933 cases. *Anaesthesia, 42*, 1316–1320.

Reisberg, B., Ferris, S. H., DeLeon, M. J., & Crook, T. (1982). The global deterioration scale for assessment of primary degenerative dementia. *American Journal of Psychiatry, 139*(9), 1136–1139.

Seeman, I. (1992). National Mortality Followback Survey. Hyattsville, MD.

Slomka, J. (1995). What do apple pie and motherhood have to do with feeding tubes and caring for the patient? *Archives of Internal Medicine, 155*, 1258–1263.

Solomon, M. Z., O'Donnell, L., Jennings, B., Guilfoy, V., Wolf, S. M., Nolan, K., Jackson, R., Kochweser, D., & Donnelly, S. (1993). Decisions near the end of life: Professional views on life-sustaining treatment. *American Journal of Public Health, 8*(1), 14–23.

Truog, R. D., & Hickey, P. R. (1991). Should newborns receive analgesics for pain? *Journal of Clinical Ethics, 2*(2), 115–116.

U.S. Department of Health and Human Services. (1992). *National mortality follow-back survey* (DHHS Publication No. 92-1856).

Vachon, M. L. S. (1994). Emotional problems in palliative medicine: Patient, family, and profession. In D. Doyle, G. Hanks, and N. MacDonald (Eds.), *Oxford Textbook of Palliative Medicine* (pp. 577–604). New York: Oxford University Press.

World Health Organization. (1990). *Cancer pain relief and palliative care.* Technical Report Services 804. Geneva: World Health Organization.

Zerwekh, J. V. (1983). The dehydration question. *Nursing '83*, 47–51.

Zerwekh, J. V. (1987). Should fluid and nutritional support be withheld from terminally ill patients? *American Journal of Hospice Care, 4*(4), 37–38.

Zerwekh, J. V. (1997). Do dying patients really need IV fluids? *American Journal of Nursing, 97*(4), 37–38.

5

Study Methods

This chapter describes the methodology of the educational component of the project. Included here is a description of the sample, the materials used, the intervention, and the data analysis.

THE SAMPLE

A total of 619 CNAs participated in this project, with 346 assigned to the intervention group and 273 to the control group. Subjects were chosen by administrative staff in nursing homes randomly selected from the 1995 *Directory of Nursing Homes.* A letter explaining the project was sent to each facility administrator, with a follow-up telephone call several weeks later. If there was no response from the administrator, an additional two follow-up calls were made before the facility was dropped from the sample. The primary reason for dropping a facility from the sample was lack of response from the administrator, but there were a few outright refusals. In those cases, the primary reason given was facility construction.

The first 100 subjects were assigned to the intervention group, and subsequent assignment to that group was random. A third sample was drawn when it became evident that additional subjects were needed in the control group to be closer in size to the intervention group. CNAs from the same nursing home were collectively assigned to either the control or intervention group. This was to ensure that subjects in the control group were not affected by any changes that might have occurred due to the intervention.

All participating nursing homes were located in New York or New Jersey, and all were within a 100 mile radius of New York City. A total of 28 facilities participated in this project (See TABLE 5.1). Eighteen of the homes were located in New York, and the remaining ten facilities were in New Jersey. The majority (16 facilities) were in urban areas, although the cities ranged in size from very large (New York City) to rather small (Passaic, NJ). Nine of the facilities were in suburban areas, and only three were rural.

Nationally, approximately two-thirds of all nursing homes are proprietary (Strahan, 1997). However, New York State has an unusually high number of not-for-profit homes. This most likely accounts for the proportionally high number of this type of facility in our sample. Half the participating facilities were not-for-profit, 13 were proprietary homes, and one facility in New Jersey was county-run.

Ten of the facilities in the project identified themselves as being religiously affiliated. Of these, four were Jewish and six were Catholic. Of the six Catholic facilities, three were

TABLE 5.1   Characteristics of Participating Facilities

Characteristics	Number of Facilities	Percent of Total
State		
New York	18	64%
New Jersey	10	36%
Facility Setting		
Urban	16	57%
Suburban	9	32%
Rural	3	11%
Profit Status		
Not for Profit	14	50%
Proprietary	13	46%
County Facility	1	4%
Religious Affiliation		
Catholic	6	21%
Jewish	4	14%
No Religious affiliation	18	64%
Number of Beds		
Less than 101	2	8%
101–200	13	46%
201–300	5	18%
301–400	3	11%
401–500	0	0%
501–600	4	14%
601–700	0	0%
701–800	1	4%

run by the Carmelite Sisters of the Aged and Infirm. The size of the participating facilities spanned a wide range, with the smallest facility having 94 beds and the largest 786. About half the facilities (15) had 200 beds or less.Each facility was asked to have as many CNAs as possible participate in the program. In general, all of the participating facilities seemed eager for their CNAs to take part in the program. However, issues of coverage, as well as varying degrees of enthusiasm and energy, influenced the number of participants. In some facilities, CNAs were selected for participation, while other nursing homes asked for volunteers. Subjects-per-facility ranged from a low of five to a high of 56, with a median number of 19. There was no relationship between size of the facility and number of participating CNAs. Interestingly, one of the smallest facilities (111 beds) had the second largest number of subjects (50).

With respect to demographic characteristics (see TABLE 5.2), the majority of CNAs (94%) were female. Their ages ranged from under 20 (1%) to over 60 (6%), with the greatest number (35%) stating they were between 40 and 49 years of age. The largest proportion of CNAs were Caribbean-born (38%) or were born in the mainland United States (38%), with an additional 4 percent coming from Puerto Rico. With respect to religion, nearly half (49%) were Protestant, while about one-third (35%) were Catholic.

TABLE 5.2   Sociodemographic Characteristics of CNAs

	n (%)
Age: (n=587)	
under 20	4 (.7)
20 to 29	80 (13.6)
30 to 39	158 (26.9)
40 to 49	206 (35.1)
50 to 59	105 (17.9)
over 59	34 (5.5)
Sex: (n=590)	
female	552 (93.6)
male	38 (6.4)
Place of Birth: (n=558)	
Asia	24 (4.3)
Africa	43 (7.7)
Caribbean	214 (38.4)
Central America	8 (1.4)
Europe	18 (3.2)
South America	22 (3.9)
United States	209 (37.5)
Puerto Rico	20 (3.6)
Religion: (n=575)	
Protestant	306 (53.2)
Catholic	202 (35.1)
Moslem	13 (2.3)
Hindu	7 (1.2)
Buddhist	2 (0.3)
No Religious Affiliation	12 (2.1)
Other	33 (5.8)

When asked how long they had been employed as CNAs, less than three percent had worked for less than one year, while a similar number worked for more than 30 years. The mean number of years employed as a CNA was 10.63 (S.D. 7.96), while the median was 8 years. Contrary to popular belief, CNAs' employment in their current job was relatively lengthy. While about eight percent were employed in their current facility less than one year, ten percent were employed in the same place for more than 20 years. The mean length of employment in the current job was 8.27 years (S.D. 7.28), while the median was 6.00. Slightly more than half (55.3%) always worked the day shift, while another 25.6 percent said they always worked the evening shift. Only 2.6% were night shift workers[1]. The remaining subjects (16.5%) worked varying shifts.

---

[1]As a rule, we did not include night shift workers because of the logistical difficulties associated with conducting sessions at night. One facility held its night inservices at 6:00 AM, so in that case we agreed to have the night shift participate. Additionally, a few facilities scheduled night shift CNAs to participate in day and evening sessions.

MATERIALS

PRETEST: ETHICS QUESTIONNAIRE

The instrument used to assess nursing assistants' knowledge and attitudes regarding ethical issues and end-of-life decision-making was a modification of a questionnaire developed by the Education Development Center (EDC) in Newton, Massachusetts, for the Decisions Near the End of Life program (Solomon et al., 1993). This instrument was originally designed for use with professional health care providers. For the purposes of the present study the questionnaire was slightly revised to be more applicable for use by a CNA population.

A readability analysis was conducted on the questionnaire at three levels: the individual item level, subsets of items, and the entire questionnaire. This analysis assured that the questions were understandable to the nursing assistants. Three readability scores were computed at each level of analysis: a Flesch Reading Ease Score, a Gunning's Fog Index, and a Flesch-Kincaid Grade Level. The Flesch Reading Ease Score determines the reading difficulty and associated grade level of text. The Gunning's Fox Index computes the appropriate grade level a reader must have achieved to understand a text, and the Flesch-Kinkaid Grade Level computes a grade level reading index as well. The use of three indices allowed us to fine-tune the readability (and thus lexic comprehensibility) of individual and subsets of items, as well as the entire questionnaire. All text determined to be at too high a reading level was revised. The questionnaire had been piloted at The Jewish Home in an earlier project, and was modified for this project after the readability analysis.

The ethics questionnaire covered several conceptual areas, including knowledge about advance directives, attitudes towards end of life decision making and care, barriers to the best possible end-of-life care, and the CNA as part of the health care team. The questionnaire also contained items pertaining to the demographics and work experience of the CNAs and a job satisfaction scale.

Knowledge About Advance Directives

The first section of the ethics questionnaire examined CNAs' general knowledge about advance directives. Specifically, subjects were asked about the types of decisions that can be made by health care agents as well as the decision-making authority of a living will. This section contained eight items, an example of which was: "If a resident left instructions (made out a living will) that she would not want to have any amputations -can the doctor perform an amputation if the resident gets gangrene?" Subjects could respond "yes," "no," or "don't know" to each of the items.

Attitudes Towards End-of-Life Treatment Decision-Making and Care

The second section of the questionnaire examined CNAs' attitudes towards care of the dying and end-of-life decision-making. Questions on patient autonomy, termination of life-sustaining treatment such as feeding tubes and antibiotics, comfort care, and truth-telling were included. Examples of these items included the following statements: "all residents who are able to make decisions for themselves have the right to refuse life-saving treatment, even if refusing such treatment may result in death," "it is possible to prevent a dying resident from feeling much pain," and "if you talk to a resident about a DNR (Do Not Resuscitate Order) they will think their condition is hopeless." For the majority of items subjects were asked to respond "agree," "disagree," or "don't know." On the remaining items subjects were asked to answer "yes" or "no." Subjects were told that almost all of these questions had no right or wrong answer; rather, they are examining CNAs' feelings towards different issues.

Three additional sub-components of CNA attitudes were examined. These included beliefs about who should make decisions for cognitively impaired residents, barriers to care, and CNAs as part of the health care team.

A.   Beliefs About Who Should Make Decisions for Cognitively Impaired Residents

Five items examined CNAs' beliefs about who is the best person to make end-of-life treatment decisions for cognitively impaired residents. CNAs were asked whether they felt "the doctor is the best person to make decisions for the resident" and whether they felt "a family member is the best person to make decisions for the residents." Subjects could indicate "agree," "disagree," or "don't know" in response to each of the items. The items were not mutually exclusive and therefore subjects could theoretically indicate that they agreed or disagreed with both items. Two additional questions examined who CNAs felt "most often makes decisions for cognitively impaired residents who might need to be fed by feeding tube and IVs" as well as who they feel "should make decisions" in these situations. In response to each of these questions subjects were instructed to circle "the doctor," "the family," or "someone else." Subjects were told they could circle more than one response if desired. Subjects were also asked whether they felt families should be able "to make decisions about treatment when there is no health care proxy and no living will." Subjects could respond "yes" or "no" to this question.

B.   Barriers to Care

This section examined those things that CNAs perceived as preventing residents from receiving the best possible care. Eight items were listed as possible barriers to care, these included: "not enough staff," "not including all staff in decisions about care," "fear of being sued," "communication problems among staff," "communication problems with residents or their families," "differences of opinions among staff," "lack of knowledge about all the possible choices that could be made," and "how much something will cost." Subjects were instructed to indicate for each item whether it interfered with residents receiving the best possible care "not at all," "somewhat," or "very much."

C.   CNAs as Part of the Health Care Team

Three items were included to determine CNAs' feelings concerning staff support and their own position within the heath care team. The first item examined whether CNAs "feel their opinions are respected by the people they work with." Subjects were requested to respond "disagree," "agree," or "don't know" to this question. Next they were asked whether they receive "support when caring for dying residents" to which they were instructed to respond: "always or almost always," "sometimes," "never or almost never," or "don't know." Lastly, they were asked how satisfied they are in their interactions with other staff members including physicians, nurses, social workers, administrators, and clergy, as well as residents, and residents' family members. Subjects responded "not satisfied," "somewhat satisfied," or "very satisfied" to each of these questions. (See Appendix A for all of the knowledge and attitude items on the Ethics Questionnaire.)

D.   Job Satisfaction

The last section of the ethics questionnaire contained an overall job satisfaction scale used with paraprofessional home care workers (Cantor & Chichin, 1990). Subjects were presented with a series of 23 items and asked to indicate on a four point Likert scale ranging from (1) "very true" to (4) "not true at all." The responses to all of the items were added together to form a global job satisfaction score, with lower scores indicating greater levels of job satisfaction.

POSTTEST: ETHICS QUESTIONNAIRE

Subjects also completed a posttest questionnaire. This contained a slightly shortened version of the ethics questionnaire. A few questions were removed in an effort to reduce the time burden on the facilities. The questions that were removed were primarily repetitive attitude questions and questions concerning barriers to care. Following the posttest, subjects again completed the overall job satisfaction scale. (See Appendix A for all of the knowledge and attitude items on the Ethics Questionnaire.)

Ethics Education Evaluation Form

At the end of the intervention, subjects in the experimental group were asked to complete a short evaluation form assessing the ethics education program. The form contained ten close-ended questions. Subjects were asked to indicate on a Likert scale ranging from (1) "not at all" to (5) "very much" how they felt about each of the questions. Higher scores indicated a more positive assessment of the program. The questionnaire also contained five open-ended questions in which subjects were asked to describe in more detail their feelings about the program. (See Appendix B for a copy of the Ethics Education Evaluation Form.)

THE INTERVENTION

Subjects who were assigned to the intervention group participated in three one-hour educational/discussion sessions. These were held within the various nursing homes generally one or two weeks apart. However, this occasionally varied, depending on the scheduling needs of the facilities. The size of the groups participating in the sessions ranged from three to twenty CNAs.

The educational/discussion sessions had a semi-structured format. The sessions were tailored to each respective facility based on how the CNAs from that facility responded to the questions on the ethics questionnaire. At each facility, the results from the pretest for that facility were presented to the CNAs. The CNAs were then encouraged to talk in more detail about the reasons for the answers they had given, their feelings in general about the various topics, as well as their own experiences caring for dying residents. Educational information about patient autonomy, advance directives, and comfort care was provided for the CNAs and was incorporated into the general discussion.

PROCEDURE

In the first session subjects in both the intervention and control groups were given an overview of the project and told that they would be participating in an ethics education program specifically for CNAs. Subjects were also told that at the end of the program they would receive a certificate for completing the ethics education program. All subjects were then given the pretest questionnaire to complete. Subjects were told not to write their names on the questionnaires and that all responses to the questionnaire and comments during the sessions would remain confidential. In order to match pretest questionnaires with posttest questionnaires that would be completed at a later date, subjects were asked to provide three pieces of information on both questionnaires: the month they were born, the first two digits of their social security number, and the last number of the year they were born. The pretest took about 45 minutes to complete.

Following the pretest, three educational sessions were scheduled for the nursing homes in the intervention group. These sessions usually began about two weeks after the pretest session. The posttest was then administered approximately six months after the last educational session.

Nursing homes that were in the control group did not receive the educational intervention between the pretest and the posttest. However, it was expected that they would continue with their usual program of inservices. In these cases, the posttest was scheduled approximately three months after the pretest. Following the posttest, subjects in the control group received a condensed one hour educational session.

ANALYSIS

Descriptive statistics, including means and frequency distributions, were conducted on the pretest data to determine CNAs' general knowledge and attitudes towards end-of-life decision-making issues.

To determine the factors related to knowledge and attitudes in end-of life decision-making, we conducted non-parametric tests for continuous variables, chi-square tests for categorical data, and multivariate logistic regression analyses. For these bivariate and multivariate analyses only those subjects who responded "disagree" (0) or "agree" (1) to the particular question were included (subjects who responded "don't know" or had missing data for that question were not included in these analyses).

The nine independent variables entered into the model were the same for all regression analyses. These variables fell into three categories: cultural and demographic characteristics of the CNA, the CNAs' work experience, and characteristics of the nursing home. (1) *Age:* The age of the CNA. This was a dichotomous variable (0=39 years of age and under; 1=40 years of age and above). (2) *wBorn:* The country in which the CNA was born. For the purposes of the logistic regression analysis this variable was divided into two categories, the United States versus all other countries (0=United States; 1=all other countries). (3) *Religion:* The importance of religion to the CNA (0=not at all important or somewhat important; 1=very important). (4) *Experience:* Whether the CNA had previous experience with cases in which residents or a health care agent refused life sustaining treatment (0=had previous experience; 1=no previous experience). (5) *yrCNA:* The number of years the subject has worked as a CNA. (6) *Job satisfaction (Jobsat):* This was a continuous variable with lower scores indicating greater job satisfaction. (7) & (8) *Religious Affiliation:* The religious affiliation of the facility in which the CNA works. As discussed above all of the facilities fell into one of three categories, Jewish, Catholic, and non-affiliated. Religious affiliation was therefore dummy coded into two variables (*Jewish:* 0=non-Jewish facility, 1=Jewish Facility; and *Catholic:* 0=non-Catholic facility, 1=Catholic facility) and entered into the logistic regression. Non-affiliated facilities, also coded as 0 and 1, were not entered into the logistic regression equation. Thus, Jewish and Catholic nursing homes were compared to non-religiously affiliated facilities. (9) *State:* The state where the nursing home was located (0=New York; 1=New Jersey).

Chi-square tests were conducted to examine changes in knowledge and attitudes from the pretest to the posttest. Two by two tables of group (control vs. experimental) by response (agree vs. disagree) were constructed for each of the items on the ethics questionnaire to determine whether there were significant differences between groups before and after the intervention. (Subjects who responded "don't know" or had missing data for the particular question analyzed were not included in the analysis.)

REFERENCES

Cantor, M., & Chichin, E. R. (1990). *Stress and strain among homecare workers of the frail elderly.* New York: Brookdale Research Institute, Third Age Center, Fordham University.

Directory of Nursing Homes. (1995). Phoenix, AZ: Oryz Press.

Solomon, M. Z., O'Donnell, L., Jennings, B., Guilfoy, V., Wolf, S. M., Nolan, K., Jackson, R., Koch-Weser, D., & Donnelly, S. (1993). Decisions near the end of life: Professional views on life-sustaining treatment. *American Journal of Public Health, 8*(2), 14–23.

Strahan, G. W. (1997). *An overview of nursing homes and their current residents: Data from the 1995 National Nursing Home Survey.* Centers for Disease Control and Prevention, U.S. Department of Health and Human Services.

6

Study Results

This chapter describes the findings from the pre and posttest questionnaires used to assess CNAs' knowledge and attitudes about ethical issues and end-of-life decision-making.

1. OVERALL FINDINGS ON THE PRETEST ETHICS QUESTIONNAIRE

Descriptive analyses were conducted to determine CNAs' general knowledge and attitudes toward end-of-life issues.

KNOWLEDGE ABOUT ADVANCE DIRECTIVES

As noted earlier, all subjects (N=619) completed the pretest questionnaire. Findings with respect to knowledge about specific issues related to end-of-life decision-making varied. (Refer to Appendix A for frequencies to all knowledge and attitude questions on the ethics questionnaire.) Subjects were more likely to correctly answer what health care agents could do, rather than what they could not do. Over 50 percent correctly answered questions about antibiotics (55%), amputations (59%), and stopping (56%) or not starting (60%) a feeding tube. On the other hand, only 41% correctly stated that a health care agent could not sell a person's home, and even fewer (21%) knew the agent could not make financial decisions.

With respect to living wills, subjects fared better. Nearly eight out of ten (79%) knew that a doctor could not legally amputate a limb if the person had a living will stating he/ she would not want an amputation. A similar proportion (83%) knew a doctor could not legally insert a feeding tube if this had been stipulated in a living will.

Interesting differences became apparent when the CNAs were divided into two groups based on whether their nursing home was located in New York or New Jersey. These differences were most evident with respect to knowledge items focusing on health care proxies and living wills. While both states have health care proxy laws, and assumedly staff in health care facilities receive inservices about these laws and advance directives, the CNAs in New York were more knowledgeable about specific aspects related to implementing these directives (see TABLE 6.1). For example, when asked if a health care agent could ask a doctor to discontinue a feeding tube once it was already in place, only half the CNAs in New Jersey knew the correct response. In contrast, nearly two-thirds of the New York CNAs knew the correct response (X^2=10.68; p=.001). Similarly, about half the New Jersey CNAs knew whether a health care agent can tell the doctor not to give a resident antibiotics when the resident has pneumonia, while 60 percent of their New York counterparts knew the correct answer (X^2=4.46; p<.05). When asked if a health care agent could sign permission for an amputation if the resident has gangrene, slightly more that two-thirds of the New York CNAs knew the correct response, while only about 56 percent of New Jersey CNAs knew the right answer (X^2=6.72; p<.01). New York CNAs were also correct more often (68% vs. 57%) concerning the health care agent's right to ask the doctor not to start a tube feeding (X^2=6.29; p<.05).

ATTITUDES ABOUT ETHICAL ISSUES AT THE END OF LIFE

In general, CNAs felt overwhelmingly that residents have the right to make treatment decisions. In response to the statement, "All residents who are able to make decisions for themselves have the right to refuse life-saving treatment, even if refusing such treatment may result in death," nearly nine out of ten CNAs (88%) chose the "agree" category. Similarly, most subjects (79%) agreed that if a resident does not want antibiotics and wants to die, or does not want a feeding tube and wants to die (83%), the nursing home should not force the treatment upon the person. In apparent contradiction, while the CNAs might agree that treatments such as feeding tubes and IVs should not be forced upon a resident, approximately half seem to feel that it is wrong not to start (49%) or to stop (55%) a feeding tube if it means the person will die. Responses to this question varied widely by facility, ranging from a high of 90 percent in one facility where CNAs felt it was okay not

TABLE 6.1   Differences Between States on Knowledge Questions (X^2 analysis)

Question	% Correct				
	New York	New Jersey	X^2	Sig. Level	N
Can a health care agent tell the doctor not to give the resident antibiotics when the resident has pneumonia? (yes)	60.7%	51.9%	4.46	.035	592
Can a health care agent ask the doctor to stop a feeding tube once it has already begun? (yes)	63.6%	50.0%	10.68	.001	595
Can a health care agent ask the doctor not to start a tube feeding if the resident is no longer taking food by mouth? (yes)	67.5%	57.2%	6.29	.012	585
Can a health care agent sign permission for an amputation if the resident has gangrene? (yes)	66.4%	55.8%	6.72	.009	589

Note: Percentages indicate the percent of subjects in New York and New Jersey that correctly answered each of the knowledge questions. No significant differences were found on the remaining knowledge questions.

to start a feeding tube, to a low of 0 percent who felt it was acceptable. Most CNAs seemed to feel there was little difference between withholding (not starting) and withdrawing (stopping) a treatment such as feeding tube or intravenous therapy. However, in almost every facility slightly fewer CNAs felt it was permissible to stop a feeding tube rather than not start it.

CNAs had mixed emotions about artificial nutrition and hydration. When asked if they felt we make dying residents more uncomfortable by giving them feeding tubes and IVs than if we don't feed them, 42 percent responded in the affirmative (although this ranged from 0 percent to 90 percent at the different facilities). More than half (56%) felt that we make dying residents more uncomfortable by continuing to give them food and water by mouth than if we didn't feed them. On the other hand, 52% said they felt a dying person should always be offered food and water by mouth, while 62% said a dying person should always receive food and water, even if by feeding tube if necessary.

CNAs were split with respect to their feelings about whether some of the treatments we give residents are too uncomfortable (40% agreeing while 44% disagree and 13% are unsure). As far as keeping dying residents free from pain, only about two-thirds (63%) think it is possible to prevent dying patients from feeling much pain. And, with respect to the principle of double effect, only about half (53%) feel it is right to give pain medication to relieve suffering if it may make the person die sooner. Interestingly, this ranged from a low of 12 percent at one of the Catholic facilities (of note because the principle of double effect has historically been invoked by the Catholic Church [Beauchamp & Childress, 1989]) to a high of 93 percent in a facility without religious auspices.

CNAs' beliefs about the extent to which nursing homes met residents' spiritual needs was also examined. It was anticipated that the facilities under religious auspices would have higher proportions of CNAs responding positively to this item[2]. In three out of five of the Catholic facilities, at least 75 percent of the CNAs felt that spiritual needs were met. Jewish facilities fared less well, with less than two-thirds of the CNAs in those facilities stating they felt spiritual needs were met. Surprisingly, in five of the non-religiously affiliated facilities more than 75% of the CNAs felt that the spiritual needs of residents received sufficient attention.

There seems to be a general belief that residents should be protected, and evidence of paternalism was apparent when it came to issues of truth-telling. Of particular note were the 70 percent of CNAs who felt that in cases where a family member asked us not to tell a resident who can understand that he/she has an illness and a certain amount of time to live, we should go along with the family's request and not tell the resident. There was, however, a great deal of variability between nursing homes in response to this item. With respect to decision-making for residents, about half the CNAs (52%) said they believe that many patients prefer to let other people make decisions for them.

A. *Beliefs About Who Should Make Decisions for Cognitively Impaired Residents*

When asked who should make treatment decisions for cognitively impaired residents, CNAs favored the families. Seventy-three percent of CNAs agreed that a family member is the

---

[2]CNAs were asked to respond to the item, "The spiritual needs of dying residents receive too little attention." The proportion who chose the "disagree" response were thought to feel that residents' spiritual needs received sufficient attention.

best person to make treatment decisions for cognitively impaired residents, while only 40 percent agreed that the doctor is the best person (these two items were not mutually exclusive; therefore, percentages could add up to be greater than 100). Additionally, more than four-fifths (82%) of the CNAs felt the family should be able to make end-of-life decisions even when there is no advance directive to guide them. Some felt very strongly about the primacy of the family, with about 30 percent of the CNAs reporting they felt families should be able to overrule residents who are able to make decisions for themselves. (For example, if a resident has pneumonia and asks not to be treated with antibiotics, families should be able to have this request disregarded.)

In their respective nursing homes, 39 percent of the CNAs reported that they believed the family made treatment decisions for mentally impaired residents who might need feeding tubes or intravenous therapy, while 34 percent said they felt the doctor made those decisions, and 20 percent reported that the doctor and the family made these decisions together. When asked who *should* make these decisions, CNAs' responses changed only slightly (42% family, 32% doctor, and 18% both family and doctor). Although these responses indicate less of a preference for family decision-making than those stated above, during the discussion sessions those CNAs who said the family and doctor should make decisions together typically felt the family was entitled to have the final say about treatment.

B. Barriers to Good Care

Attempts were made to ascertain what CNAs perceive to be barriers to good care. The two areas that were most often rated by CNAs as being "very much a problem" were "not enough staff" (39% of the time) and "fear of lawsuits" (32% of the time). The next two items most frequently reported to be "very much a problem" were related to the transmission of information among staff. These were "communication problems among staff" (27%) and "not including all staff in decisions about treatment" (25%).

C. Role of the CNA Within the Health Care Team

A number of questions focused on the role of the CNA within the health care team. Less than half of the CNAs (46%) said their opinions about what should be done for residents were valued by the people with whom they work. In discussions during the educational sessions, however, many CNAs said they felt their opinions were valued by other CNAs. It was other members of the health care team whom they felt disregarded them and their views.

This perception was corroborated by another question that asked how satisfied CNAs were with their conversations with other staff members, as well as with residents and with families. Included in the list of staff were doctors, nurses, social workers, clergy, and administrators. CNAs were most satisfied with the conversations they had with nurses about resident care and resident conditions, with only 16% reporting they were not satisfied with these conversations. CNAs were most dissatisfied with conversations with administrators (40% not at all satisfied); this was felt to be partly a function of the minimal conversations CNAs typically have with this level of staff. Discussions with physicians were also not rated highly, with 39% saying they were not at all satisfied. When this subject was introduced in the educational sessions, many CNAs reported that they were not permitted to talk to doctors about the residents, and the only thing that doctors asked them was where a chart might be located, or where a resident might be if she was not in her room.

Surprisingly, conversations with social workers were not particularly satisfying. Thirty percent of the CNAs said they were not at all satisfied with their conversations with social workers. Also surprising, given the number of residents who die in nursing homes, was that 42 percent of CNAs reported that nursing assistants who are caring for residents who are dying never or almost never get emotional support or counseling. In three facilities, no CNAs chose the always or almost always response, and the highest proportion of CNAs who chose this response in any one nursing home was fifty percent. In one facility, 90 percent of the CNAs reported that they never received emotional support.

2.   CNAS' PERSONAL CHARACTERISTICS AND THEIR VIEWS ON END-OF-LIFE ISSUES

We had hypothesized that there might be some differences in how CNAs felt about end-of-life issues based on a number of their personal characteristics. Among these were how long they had been employed as a CNA, where they were born, and the importance of religion in their lives. Accordingly, we looked at the relationships between these variables and several of the items assessing attitudes.

A. YEARS OF EXPERIENCE AS A CNA AND ATTITUDES ABOUT END-OF-LIFE ISSUES

In order to ascertain whether there was a difference in attitudes between those who are employed for different lengths of time, we looked at the relationship between years of experience and responses to specific items on the pretest (see TABLE 6.2). The responses indicated that subjects who worked as CNAs for longer periods of time were more in favor of feeding tubes and IVS, while those who had less experience favored trying to feed by mouth. When we asked CNAs whether they felt that sometimes it is right to stop a treatment, such as a feeding tube, even if it means the person might die sooner, subjects who agreed with this had worked for significantly less time as CNAs (median=8 years) than subjects who disagreed (median=9 years; p<.05).

Subjects who agreed with the statement, "a dying person should always be offered food and water by mouth" worked for significantly less time (median=8 years) than CNAs who disagreed (median=10; p<.01). On the other hand, when we asked if CNAs felt we make dying residents more uncomfortable by continuing to give them food and water by mouth than if we didn't, those who agreed had worked significantly longer as CNAs (median=9 years) than those who disagreed (median=8 years).

Differences in length of work experience were also found in the view equating not treating with assisted suicide. Subjects who agreed that "letting a patient die by not giving them a certain treatment is the same thing as helping them to commit suicide" had worked longer as CNAs (median=9 years) than those who disagreed (median=7 years; p<.01).

There seems to be a relationship between length of employment and feeling somewhat paternalistic. For example, when CNAs were asked if a resident was suffering from some condition that causes him or her to be unable to make a decision, those who agreed that

TABLE 6.2   Years of Experience as CNA by Attitude Questions

Question	Years of Experience		
	Disagree Median	Agree Median	p
Sometimes it is right to *stop* a treatment, such as a feeding tube, even if it means a resident may die sooner.	9.00	8.00	.042
A dying person should always be offered food and water by mouth.	10.00	8.00	.003
Sometimes we make dying residents more uncomfortable by continuing to give them food and water by mouth than if we didn't.	8.00	9.00	.025
Letting a patient die by not giving them a certain treatment is the same thing as helping them to commit suicide.	7.00	9.00	.002
If a resident is suffering from some condition that causes him or her to be unable to make a decision (for example, Alzheimer's disease), the *doctor* is the best person to make decisions for the resident.	8.00	10.00	.004
I am not comfortable caring for residents who will most likely die because *their health care proxies* are refusing life-sustaining treatment.	8.00	10.00	.006
If a resident does not want antibiotics and wants to die, the nursing home should not force the treatment upon the resident.	11.00	8.00	.019
If a family asks us not to tell a resident, *who can understand,* that he or she has an illness and a certain amount of time to live, we should go along with the family's request and not tell the resident.	7.00	9.00	.002

Note: Scores indicate the mean number of years experience of CNAs who responded "agree" or "disagree" on each question. No significant differences were found on the remaining attitude questions.

the doctor was the best person to make the decision had worked for a median of ten years, while those who disagreed worked for a median of eight years (p<.01). Similarly, when asked to respond to the statement, "I am not comfortable caring for residents who will most likely die because their health care proxies are refusing life-sustaining treatment," those who agreed had worked for more time (median=10 years) than those who disagreed (median=8; p<.01).

B.   DIFFERENCES OF OPINION BETWEEN U.S.-BORN SUBJECTS AND ALL OTHER SUBJECTS

Anecdotal evidence had suggested to us that CNAs from different countries may feel differently about some of the issues we were exploring than CNAs who were U.S.-born (see TABLE 6.3). Accordingly, we compared all the CNAs born on the United States mainland with CNAs who listed their place of birth as any place other than the mainland U.S. Statistically significant differences between these two groups were found by Chi-square analysis in a number of areas.

With respect to questions related to treatment and patient autonomy, U.S.-born subjects were significantly more pro-autonomy than their non-U.S.-born counterparts. When asked

TABLE 6.3   Attitude Questions by Country of Birth (X^2 analysis)

Question	% Agree		X^2	Sig.	N
	USA	Non-USA			
Sometimes it is right *not to start* a treatment, such as a feeding tube, even if it means a resident may die sooner.	54.9%	34.5%	19.41	.000	480
Sometimes it is right to *stop* a treatment, such as a feeding tube, even if it means a resident may die sooner.	45.0%	30.3%	10.52	.001	480
A dying person should always receive food and water, even by feeding tube if necessary.	61.2%	73.6%	8.57	.003	510
Letting a patient die by not giving him/her a certain treatment is the same thing as helping him/her commit suicide.	48.6%	67.3%	16.62	.000	492
Some residents or their families have sued doctors when the residents were given a treatment to keep them alive that they did not want.	86.7%	77.7%	5.03	.025	414
Discontinuing a feeding tube is the same as killing a resident.	30.3%	42.1%	6.86	.009	489
Many patients prefer not to know they are dying.	74.2%	86.9%	12.72	.000	498
In this nursing home the spiritual needs of dying residents receive too little attention.	41.4%	30.7%	5.71	.017	482
I am not comfortable caring for residents who will most likely die because they are refusing life-sustaining treatment.	11.0%	24.6%	14.44	.000	509

Note: Percentages presented indicate the percent of subjects that "agree" with each of the attitude questions. No significant differences were found for the remaining questions.

if "sometimes it is right not to start a treatment, such as a feeding tube, even if it means the person may die sooner," 54.9 percent of the U.S.-born CNAs agreed, while only 34.5 percent of the other CNAs agreed (X^2=12.41; p<.001). In response to the statement, "Sometimes it is right to stop a treatment, such as a feeding tube, even if it means a resident may die sooner," 45.0 percent of the U.S.-born CNAs agreed, while only 30.3 percent of the others agreed (X^2=10.52; p<.001).

Similar differences were found when questions about comfort were asked. When asked if a dying person should always receive food and water, even if by feeding tube if necessary, 61.2% of the U.S.-born CNAs agreed, while 73.6% of the non-U.S.-born agreed (X^2=8.57; p<.003). U.S.-born CNAs were more likely (41.4%) than non-U.S.-born CNAs (30.7%) to agree that the spiritual needs of dying residents receive too little attention (X^2=5.71, p<05).

When confronted with the statement, "Letting a patient die by not giving him/her a certain treatment is the same thing as helping him/her to commit suicide," about half (48.6%) of the U.S.-born CNAs agreed, while two-thirds (67.3%) of the other CNAs agreed (X^2=16.62; p<.001). Similarly, when asked if discontinuing a feeding tube is the same as killing a patient, only 30.3% of the U.S.-born CNAs agreed, while 42.4% of the non-U.S.-born CNAs agreed (X^2=6.86; p<.01).

Non-U.S.-born CNAs were less comfortable caring for residents who are dying because they are refusing life-sustaining treatment than were U.S.-born CNAs (24.6% vs. 11.0%; X^2=14.44; p<.001). Both groups were less comfortable caring for residents who were dying because their health care agents refused life-sustaining treatment (20.7% U.S.-born; 28.4% non-U.S.-born). However, there were no significant differences between the two groups. Non-U.S.-born CNAs were also more likely than their U.S. counterparts to believe that many patients prefer not to know that they are dying (86.9% vs. 74.2%; X^2=12.72; p<.001).

Finally, U.S.-born CNAS (86.7%) were more likely than other CNAs (77.7%) to agree that doctors have been sued for overtreating (X^2=5.03; p<.05).

C. Religiosity and Attitudes About End-of-Life Care

Another area we felt might be associated with how CNAs felt about end-of-life issues was the degree to which they felt religion is important in their lives (see TABLE 6.4). CNAs were divided into two groups, those who said that religion was not important or only somewhat important to them, and those who stated that religion was very important. For many of the items related to attitudes about end-of-life care, the responses of these two groups differed significantly. For example, in response to whether it is right not to start a feeding tube, even if the patient may die sooner, more than half (56.2%) of the less religious agreed with the statement, while slightly more than one-third (38.3%) of those who described themselves as very religious felt that way (X^2=9.64; p<.01). Slightly more than half (53.8%) of the less religious felt that a dying person should always receive food and water, even if by feeding tube if necessary, while nearly three quarters (71.4%) of the very religious thought this should happen (X^2=10.74; p=.001).

More than 40 percent of the more religious (41.1%) felt that discontinuing a feeding tube is killing a patient, while only about 20 percent of the less religious felt that way (X^2=12.11; p=.001). About two-thirds (66.4%) of the very religious felt that letting a patient die by not giving them a feeding tube is the same thing as helping them commit suicide, while only about one-third (36.7%) of the less religious felt that way (X^2=27.56; p<.001). The less religious were more likely (65.1%) than the very religious (46.9%) to believe that we sometimes make dying residents more uncomfortable by giving them feeding tubes and IVs than if we didn't (X^2=6.55; p=.01). A greater proportion of those who identified themselves as less religious think it is right to give pain medication to relieve suffering, even if the person may die sooner (81.0% of the less religious vs. 62.5% of the more religious; X^2=10.54; p=.001).

While we found an overall tendency toward paternalism, it seemed to be more prevalent among those who described themselves as very religious. More than eight out of ten (84.1%) of the very religious believe that many patients prefer not to know they are dying, compared to 71.6 percent of the less religious (X^2=7.70; p<.01). Also, having higher regard for family wishes over a resident's right to have information was obvious. When asked if a family member asks us not to tell a resident who can understand that he/she has an illness and a certain amount of time to live, we should go along with the family's request and not tell the resident, 71.0 percent of the less religious agreed, while 81.6 percent of the more religious agreed (X^2=5.38; p<.05).

TABLE 6.4   Importance of Religion to the CNA by Attitude Towards End-of-Life Issues (X^2 analysis)

Question	Not at all or somewhat important	Very important	X^2	Sig. Level	N
	% Agreeing that religion is:				
Sometimes it is right *not to start* a feeding tube, even if the resident may die sooner.	56.2%	38.3%	9.64	.002	504
Sometimes it is right to *stop* a feeding tube, even if it means a resident may die sooner.	44.9%	33.7%	4.00	.045	501
A dying person should always receive food and water, even by feeding tube if necessary.	53.8%	71.4%	10.74	.001	538
Sometimes we make dying residents more uncomfortable by giving them feeding tubes and IVs than if we didn't feed them.	65.1%	49.6%	6.55	.010	476
If you talk to residents about a DNR (Do Not Resuscitate) order they will think their condition is hopeless.	36.4%	56.6%	11.79	.001	484
Letting a patient die by not giving them a certain treatment is the same thing as helping them to commit suicide.	36.7%	66.4%	27.56	.000	515
Discontinuing a feeding tube is the same as killing a resident.	21.7%	41.1%	12.11	.001	515
Sometimes it is right to give pain medication to relieve suffering even if it will make the person die sooner.	81.0%	62.5%	10.54	.001	489
Many patients prefer not to know they are dying.	71.6%	84.1%	7.70	.006	527
I am not comfortable caring for residents who will most likely die because *they* are refusing life-sustaining treatment.	11.7%	20.6%	3.94	.047	527
I am not comfortable caring for residents who will most likely die because *their health care agent* is refusing life-sustaining treatment.	14.4%	27.9%	7.05	.008	502
It is wrong to stop antibiotics, if it will keep the resident alive, even if the resident doesn't want it.	32.5%	45.2%	4.52	.034	481
It is wrong to stop a feeding tube, if it will keep the resident alive, even if the resident doesn't want it.	35.3%	47.8%	4.41	.036	489
If a family member asks us not to tell a resident, *who can understand*, that he/she has an illness and a certain amount of time to live we should go along with the family's request and not tell the resident.	71.0%	81.6%	5.38	.020	523

Note: No significant differences were found on the remaining attitude questions.

3.   MULTIVARIATE LOGISTIC REGRESSION ANALYSES

To examine which variables were most strongly related to CNAs' attitudes toward ethical issues in end-of-life decision-making, multivariate logistic regression analyses were conducted. The independent variables included cultural and demographic characteristics of the CNAs, the CNAs' work experience, and characteristics of the nursing home. The results suggest that CNAs' place of birth (wborn); religious importance (religion); and job satisfaction (jobsat) were key factors in predicting CNAs' attitudes towards ethical issues in end-of-life decision-making. The number of years as a CNA (yrCNA) was only associated with questions 1, 3, 6, 10 and 16. TABLE 6.5 displays the results for each question and independent variable.

4.   POSTTEST RESULTS

As noted earlier, CNAs were assigned to either an intervention group (n=346) or a control group (n=273). In the case of the control group, CNAs completed a posttest questionnaire a few months after completing the pretest, and were exposed only to whatever routine inservices they ordinarily attend. The intervention group CNAs completed the posttest approximately six months after the final educational session. (See TABLE 6.6 for a comparison of pre and posttest differences.)

KNOWLEDGE OF ADVANCE DIRECTIVES

With respect to questions assessing what CNAs know about health care proxies and living wills, there were no significant differences between the control group and the intervention groups in the pretest. In the posttest, however, there were statistically significant differences between the two groups on a number of items.

As far as non-treatment decisions (i.e., financial or legal decisions) are concerned, about two-fifths (39.1%) of the experimental group knew that a health care proxy cannot make financial decisions for the resident, as compared with only about one-fifth (22.2%; p<.001) of the control group. Similarly, more than half (54.3%) of the experimental group knew that a health care proxy cannot sell the resident's home or apartment.

After participating in the education sessions, significantly more of the experimental group knew the correct answers on treatment-related issues. For example, when asked if a health care proxy could ask the doctor not to start a feeding tube if a resident is no longer taking food by mouth, more than three quarters of the experimental group (77.1%) chose the correct response, while only 61.3 percent (p<.001) of the control group knew the right answer. In response to a question about whether a health care proxy could sign permission for an amputation if a resident had gangrene, 72.4 percent of the experimental subjects knew the correct response, in contrast to 62.9% (p<.05) of the controls. Nearly 92 percent (91.7%) of the CNAs who attended the education sessions (i.e., the experimental group) knew that a nursing home could not insert a feeding tube in a resident if that resident left instructions that he would not want to be fed by feeding tube if he could no

TABLE 6.5   Associations with CNA Agreement to the Attitude Questions[a]

Attitude Questions	Age	wBorn	Religion	Exper	yrCNA	Jobsat	Jewish	Catholic	State
1.	1.175	0.430***	0.566*	0.890	0.963*	1.003	0.705	0.679	0.968
2.	1.422	0.488**	0.650	0.860	0.968	1.019	0.558	0.969	0.836
3.	1.169	0.679	0.857	1.105	0.955**	0.996	1.199	0.733	0.820
4.	1.331	1.324	1.852*	1.294	0.971	0.990	2.003*	1.057	1.142
5.	1.880*	0.691	0.669	0.913	1.006	1.007	1.087	0.905	0.737
6.	1.422	0.544**	0.567*	0.857	0.968*	1.013	1.207	0.564*	0.926
7.	1.413	1.317	2.408**	0.948	1.013	1.015	1.174	1.255	1.864**
8.	0.739	0.381	0.000	0.635	1.044	1.020	0.861	0.645	0.650
9.	1.261	0.730	1.270	0.670	0.981	0.979*	1.627	0.998	0.853
10.	1.272	2.159**	2.944***	0.841	1.035*	0.998	1.133	1.025	1.003
11.	1.100	0.482*	0.938	0.683	1.010	1.026	0.643	0.979	0.775
12.	1.090	0.877	0.722	0.823	0.877	1.012	0.621*	0.940	1.042
13.	0.930	1.577	2.785**	1.159	1.022	0.986	1.707	1.274	1.389
14.	0.820	1.245	0.355**	0.511**	1.021	1.009	0.869	0.796	0.824
15.	0.857	2.207**	1.533	0.906	1.031	0.999	3.635*	1.082	1.652
16.	1.119	1.410	1.589	1.118	1.034*	0.984	0.773	0.583*	0.981
17.	1.095	1.774*	0.706	1.066	1.005	1.001	0.865	1.111	1.389
18.	1.084	0.868	1.194	0.686	1.004	0.988	0.584	0.959	0.932
19.	1.447	0.529**	1.595	0.748	0.999	1.041***	1.099	0.564	0.859
20.	0.970	1.057	1.939*	0.737	1.007	0.970**	1.246	1.113	0.708
21.	1.206	2.804**	2.869*	0.974	1.027	1.050***	1.585	1.557	0.854
22.	1.211	1.547	2.579*	0.868	1.051	1.048***	1.176	0.747	0.766
23.	0.752	0.801	0.958	0.688	0.990	1.042***	1.753	1.466	0.850
24.	0.599	0.995	1.331	1.224	0.994	0.999	0.942	1.003	0.741
25.	0.320**	0.755	1.143	1.611	1.030	1.000	3.019	1.630	0.679
26.	0.583	0.725	0.743	0.820	0.991	1.007	0.883	1.154	0.662
27.	0.752	0.606	0.606	0.901	0.981	1.002	0.696	0.562	0.823
28.	1.260	0.867	2.160*	1.061	1.023	1.017	1.295	0.974	1.307
29.	1.400	1.234	1.860*	1.068	1.016	1.000	1.623	0.902	1.427
30.	2.090*	0.846	1.612	1.169	1.004	0.956***	3.251**	0.892	1.805*
31.	2.320*	1.171	1.384	1.232	0.986	1.009	0.910	2.440**	1.137
32.	1.397	1.087	0.716	0.682	0.976	0.997	0.897	1.255	0.689

Note: [a] Odds ratios are presented in TABLE 6.5.
*p < .05. **p < .01. ***p < .001

Questions Pertaining to TABLE 6.5

1. Sometimes it is right *not to start* a treatment, such as a feeding tube, even if it means a resident might die sooner.
2. Sometimes it is right to *stop* a treatment, such as a feeding tube, even if it means a resident may die sooner.
3. A dying person should always be offered food and water by mouth.
4. A dying person should always receive food and water, even by feeding tube if necessary.
5. Sometimes we make dying residents more uncomfortable by continuing to give them food and water by mouth than if we didn't.
6. Sometimes we make dying residents more uncomfortable by giving them tube feedings and IVs than if we didn't feed them.
7. If you talk to a resident about a DNR (Do Not Resuscitate) order they will think their condition is hopeless.
8. All residents who are able to make decisions for themselves have the right to refuse life-saving treatment, even if refusing such treatment may result in death.
9. Many residents prefer to let people make decisions for them.
10. Letting a patient die by not giving them a certain treatment is the same thing as helping them to commit suicide.
11. Some residents or their families have sued doctors when the residents were given a treatment to keep them alive that they did not want.
12. It is possible to prevent dying residents from feeling much pain.
13. Discontinuing a feeding tube is the same as killing a resident.
14. Sometimes it is right to give pain medication to relieve suffering, even if it will make a person die sooner.
15. Many patients prefer not to know they are dying.
16. If a resident is suffering from some condition that causes him or her to be unable to make a decisions (for example, Alzheimer's disease), the *doctor* is the best person to make decisions for the resident.
17. If a resident is suffering from some condition that causes him or her to be unable to make a decisions (for example, Alzheimer's disease), a *family member* is the best person to make decisions for the resident.
18. We should not use expensive treatments to keep very old people alive.
19. In this nursing home the spiritual needs of dying residents receive too little attention.
20. My opinions about what should be done for residents are valued by the people I work with.
21. I am not comfortable caring for residents who will most likely die because *they* are refusing life-sustaining treatment.
22. I am not comfortable caring for residents who will most likely die because *their health care proxies* are refusing life-sustaining treatment.
23. Sometimes I feel the treatments we give the residents are too uncomfortable for them.
24. If a resident wants antibiotics in order to be kept alive the nursing home should provide them.
25. If a resident wants a feeding tube in order to be kept alive the nursing home should provide it.
26. If a resident does not want antibiotics and wants to die, the nursing home should not force the treatment upon the resident.
27. If a resident does not want tube feeding and wants to die, the nursing home should not force the treatment upon the resident.
28. It is wrong to stop antibiotics, if they will keep the resident alive, even if the resident doesn't want them.
29. It is wrong to stop a feeding tube, if it will keep the resident alive, even if the resident doesn't want it.
30. If a family asks us not to tell a resident, *who can understand*, that he or she has an illness and a certain amount of time to live, we should go along with the family's request and not tell the resident.
31. Do you think the family should be able to make decisions about treatment when there is no health care proxy and no living will?
32. Do you agree that when residents are capable of making decisions concerning life-threatening conditions (for example, if they have pneumonia but ask not to be treated with antibiotics), that their families should be able to overrule the resident's decision?

TABLE 6.6   Knowledge Differences Between Groups on the Pre and Posttests

Question	% Correct			
	Intervention	Control	X²	N
Can a health care proxy make financial decisions for the resident?	ªPre: 22.9% ᵇPost: 39.1%	20.7% 22.2%	.43 13.8***	597 420
Can a health care proxy tell the doctor not to give the resident antibiotics when the resident has pneumonia?	Pre: 59.2% Post: 67.7%	54.8% 59.5%	1.12 3.02⁺	592 420
Can a health care proxy sell the resident's home or apartment?	Pre: 42.0% Post: 54.3%	43.1% 41.3%	.07 6.94**	591 418
Can a health care proxy ask the doctor to stop a tube feeding once it has already begun?	Pre: 58.7% Post: 64.8%	57.9% 59.1%	.041 1.40	595 414
Can a health care proxy ask the doctor not to start a tube feeding if the resident is no longer taking food by mouth?	Pre: 65.4% Post: 77.1%	61.3% 61.3%	1.06 11.94***	585 406
Can a health care proxy sign permission for an amputation if the resident has gangrene?	Pre: 64.9% Post: 72.4%	59.0% 62.9%	2.13 4.12*	589 406
If a resident left instructions that he would not want to be fed by feeding tube if he could no longer swallow and would never regain the ability to swallow food, can the nursing home give him a feeding tube anyway?	Pre: 87.8% Post: 91.7%	81.9% 82.0%	4.04* 8.56**	600 407
If a resident left instructions that she would not want to have any amputations, can the doctor perform an amputation if the resident gets gangrene?	Pre: 83.3% Post: 83.8%	81.4% 80.9%	.369 .603	592 407

Note: ⁺ p < .1, * p < .05, ** p < .01, *** p < .001
a: pre = pretest; b: post = posttest

longer swallow and would never regain the ability to swallow. In contrast, only 82.0 percent of the control group knew the correct response to that item (p<.01).

Attitudes About End-of-Life Care and Treatment Decision-Making

Chi-square analyses were conducted to determine whether there were differences by group (intervention vs. control) on responses to the attitude questions for both the pretest and the posttest. The analyses were carried out only for those seventeen attitude questions that were included on both the pretests and posttests. (As discussed in the method section, some questions were dropped due to time constraints.)

Pretest differences between the control and intervention groups were found on two of the items. Subjects in the intervention group were more likely to "agree" (64.9%) that a dying person should always be offered food and water by mouth than subjects in the control group (49.4%; p<.001). Intervention subjects were also more likely (67.0%) than control subjects (53.9%) to "agree" that many residents prefer to let other people make decisions for them. Additionally, on the pretest more than four-fifths (85%) of the intervention group felt that family members should be able to make decisions for residents with Alzheimer's disease who are unable to make decisions for themselves. In contrast, 78 percent of the control group felt this way (p<.05). This difference was not found on the posttest with 80.4 percent of the intervention subjects and 83.2 percent of the control group (p=.481) agreeing with the statement.

Given the difficulties associated with changing attitudes, we did not anticipate that we would be able to modify the way CNAs felt about end-of-life treatment issues after participation in just three educational sessions. However, there were a number of areas where we did spend a good deal of discussion time in the sessions. Interestingly, significant differences were found in these areas after CNAs participated in the three-session educational program.

Items in which there were significant differences between the intervention and control groups were drawn from areas that included respect for autonomy and spiritual issues. When asked if letting patients die by not giving them a certain treatment is the same as helping them commit suicide, less than half (48.4%) of those CNAs that participated in the educational sessions agreed. In contrast, almost two-thirds (61.4%) of those who did not attend the sessions agreed.

In the area of respect for autonomy, both the intervention and the control groups responded similarly in the pretests when asked if they are comfortable caring for residents who will most likely die because their health care proxies are refusing life-sustaining treatment (23.7% of the intervention group; 27.2% of the control group). After attending the educational sessions, however, the proportion of the intervention group who felt uncomfortable dropped to 13.4%, as opposed to 23.8 % of the controls.

Significant differences between the intervention and control groups were also found in the area of comfort care. Subjects in the intervention group (46.6%) were significantly more likely than subjects in the control group (35.5%; p<.05) to "agree" that we sometimes give residents treatments that are too uncomfortable for them. Additionally, intervention subjects were less likely to "agree" (30.1%) than control subjects (43.0%) that the spiritual needs of dying residents receive too little attention.

REFERENCES

Beauchamp, T. L., & Childress, J. F. (1989). *Principles of biomedical ethics* 3rd ed. New York: Oxford University Press.

7

CNAs: How They See Themselves and How We Saw Them

As noted repeatedly in this volume, certified nursing assistants are key players in long term care. While care in nursing homes is provided by an interdisciplinary team consisting of a number of professional and paraprofessional members, the reality is that the bulk of hands-on care is delivered by CNAs. Given the intensity and longevity of the relationships that develop between the nursing assistant and the resident, in many instances she (or he) will become the most important person in the everyday life of the nursing home resident.

A major force behind the development of this project was our belief that CNAs are extremely valuable to the functioning of a long term care facility, and that they should be supported to the greatest extent possible. We were pleased to find this perception was shared by nearly all the administrative personnel with whom we dealt in the course of the project, and that it is increasingly becoming evident in much of the nursing home literature as well (e.g., Kane & Caplan, 1991; Libow & Starer, 1989). However, while we feel strongly that CNAs are so important, our experience in working with them prior to undertaking this project led us to believe that they did not feel that others regarded them as valuable, and we questioned how they perceived themselves. While there is some literature describing how others view CNAs (e.g., Foner, 1994; Looman, Noelker, Schur, Whitlach, & Ejaz, 1997) we were unsure as to their own opinions of their role and their value. Thus, a secondary motivation for conducting this project was to explore this in some depth. And, while we were interested in knowing how CNAs saw themselves and perceived others as seeing them, we were particularly curious about how they saw their role in their residents' end-of-life issues, as well as their view on their role within the caregiving team. Accordingly, we asked CNAs a number of questions about these issues. In an attempt to assess how they felt about what we saw as perhaps the most important job in long term care, we focused also on their opinions of their interpersonal relationships with staff and families. Another area of interest to us was the extent to which they feel they receive emotional support for the difficult work they do.

To learn how CNAs felt they were regarded by others with whom they worked, and to see the extent to which they felt they were integrated into the caregiving team, we asked them about the extent to which they were satisfied with conversations about resident care they may have had with a variety of other staff members. We also spent a good deal of time in the educational sessions discussing these conversations and how CNAs feel about them.

Sadly, as noted earlier, fewer than half the CNAs felt their opinions were respected by those with whom they work. When we attempted to elicit from them how they felt they were perceived by others in their work settings, they opined that their peers were, for the most part, respectful of their views on resident care. In general, all the other CNAs seemed to value their opinions, as did some nurses. But the sense of feeling respected essentially seemed to stop there.

When we asked the CNAs about the conversations they had about resident care with nurses, and if they were happy with the quality of these conversations, most of the CNAs reported that they were, in general, satisfied with these verbal interactions with nurses. In some facilities, however, CNAs reported that they felt they were held in low regard by nurses. Some nurses made comments such as, "Oh, you. You're just a CNA." And unfortunately, how nurses treated them was only the tip of the iceberg: they also felt that other professionals minimized the importance of the work they do. Additionally, some expressed the feeling that family members tended to hold them in low regard.

In fact, communication with families was an area about which many CNAs expressed displeasure. Apparently, it is not an uncommon practice for facility policy to prohibit CNAs from talking to families about residents' conditions. This rule was in place in a number of homes, despite the fact that CNAs spent the most time with the resident, performed for them the most intimate caregiving tasks, and clearly knew them better than any other staff member. The practice in these facilities was that the nursing assistant was required to refer the family to the nurse when asked about the resident by a family member. The nurse, of course, had to turn to the nursing assistant to obtain the necessary information about the resident's condition, and then the nurse would give that information to the family.

Frequently, the CNAs felt that referring families to the nurse was an acceptable course of action. In those cases, CNAs were relieved that the responsibility for giving any information to families was not on their shoulders. However, they were often struck by the irony of the situation: the family must ask the nurses for information about the resident, but the nurses get essentially all their information about residents' conditions from the CNAs.

EMOTIONAL SUPPORT ON THE JOB

The gerontological literature is replete with articles attesting to the burdensome aspects and strains associated with caregiving to frail elders (e.g., Cantor, 1983; Horowitz, 1985). Although most of this literature focuses on informal caregivers (i.e., families and friends), some have suggested that there are burdensome aspects of caregiving for formal (paid) caregivers as well (e.g., Cantor and Chichin, 1990; Grau, Colombotos, & Gorman, 1992). Caring for a residents who dies after one forms a close attachment with him or her is a difficult, emotionally draining experience. Doing this repeatedly, with resident after resident, could potentially become overwhelming. Thus, we were interested in the extent to which CNAs felt they received emotional support for what they do. To do this, we asked them to respond to one item in the questionnaire assessing this issue. Additionally, we spent a fair amount of time in the educational sessions focusing on emotional support.

Of note was something repeatedly told to us in almost every facility in which we conducted the project. CNAs regularly reported that they were instructed not to become "close" to the resident, the implication being that this is unprofessional. However, many CNAs also regularly told us told us that they found this impossible. As well, they considered developing relationships with residents to be a positive part of the job, and thus continued to form them.

There was quite a bit of discussion among the CNAs about the degree to which they feel they do, or do not, get emotional support on the job, particularly when caring for residents who are dying. In total, slightly less than half the CNAs feel they get support. Exploring this in the educational sessions revealed that in some cases, CNAs don't really feel they necessarily need emotional support. Many CNAs stated that this is their job, and the expectation is that they should just do it. Accordingly, the CNAs who held this view were not particularly distressed by the absence of support. In contrast, other CNAs reported that they would appreciate emotional support, and felt it would help them perform their jobs more effectively.

Interestingly, however, when looking at the responses to the questionnaire item assessing emotional support by individual nursing home, there is wide variation. The fact that absence of emotional support is an accepted feature of the job was particularly evident in one facility operated by the Carmelite Sisters. In this nursing home, CNAs were very clear about what they perceived to be one of the most important aspect of the job: care of the dying. These CNAs reported that they always sat at the bedsides of dying residents, believing that no one should die alone. They felt that support of the dying was their responsibility, and they shouldered it willingly. They stated emphatically that there was absolutely no need for them to be given emotional support for doing this.

A particularly touching story about this facility illustrates how strongly these CNAs felt about this responsibility. A newly married nursing assistant, scheduled to work the night shift, knew of a resident who was dying. Staffing that particular night was quite limited, and the nursing assistant was concerned about the resident dying by herself. Accordingly, she called her husband, a burly construction worker, to come in. He sat by the bedside of the dying resident, holding her hand until morning.

THE ROLE OF CNAS' PERSONAL CHARACTERISTICS

Clearly, CNAs are not a homogenous group, and we hypothesized that some of their personal traits might be associated with how they felt about different issues. We were particularly curious about the extent to which some of the CNAs' personal characteristics might be associated with their views on end-of-life care. Therefore, as noted in the chapter on methodology, we asked the CNAs to tell us how long they had been a CNA, and how long they were employed in the facility in which they currently worked. Additionally, since we felt ethnicity might play a role in how they perceived certain aspects of end-of-life care, we asked about their respective ethnic background. And finally, as far as personal characteristics were concerned, we thought the degree of religiosity might also be a factor in their feelings, so we asked them how religious they were.

A. LENGTH OF TIME ON THE JOB

Interestingly, the length of time an individual was employed as a nursing assistant was associated with how she (or he) felt about a number of issues. For example, those CNAs who had been employed for longer periods of time seemed to be less favorably disposed toward residents' refusing feeding tubes. They generally preferred that residents be kept alive with tubes, sometimes even if tube feeding was not consistent with the resident's wishes. These more seasoned CNAs were also more likely to feel that letting a patient die by not giving them a certain treatment was the same thing as helping them commit suicide. While we cannot be sure of the reasons for this, one possible explanation is that newer CNAs may be more aligned with respecting patient autonomy than CNAs who were trained years ago and have been employed for longer periods. As noted elsewhere in this volume, there has been a trend in health care toward the primacy of patient autonomy. This trend, which had been growing for a number of years, was legislated in 1991 with the passage of the federal Patient Self Determination Act. New CNAs, and those hired since this law was passed, are introduced to the concept of respect for patient autonomy from the beginning of their training. While most CNAs are in-serviced regularly on issues associated with residents' rights, the right to refuse life-sustaining treatment really began to assume prominence only in the past several years. All CNAs are now taught about a resident's right to accept or refuse treatment, and our responsibility to respect their choices. This concept may be more difficult for CNAs who have been on the job longer to accept.

B. THE ROLE OF CULTURE

Given our anecdotal experience with CNAs prior to conducting this project, we were curious about the extent to which cultural background might be associated with how CNAs perceived their work in general and end-of-life treatment issues in particular. As noted earlier, interesting differences were found between the CNAs who were born in the United States and those who were born in other countries. Most significant was the pro-autonomy feeling manifested by the U.S.-born CNAs, despite the fact that the United States is by no means homogeneous. Compared to the less positive feelings about autonomy expressed by those from the other countries, those from the United States were clearly more in favor of an individual's right to make his or her own decisions. While this is noteworthy, it is certainly not surprising, given the American attitudes toward independence and self-determination. Cultural attitudes toward family relationships may come into play when it comes to life in general, as well as to issues of who makes decisions, specifically. While most cultures attach importance to the family system, the strong U.S. acceptance of individual independence, in concert with the more interdependent family relationships of those born in other countries, may explain, in part, why these two groups may have different views.

Another area where there were differences among CNAs born in the U.S. and those born in other countries were issues associated with feeding. The non-U.S.-born CNAs had stronger feelings than the U.S.-born about giving dying residents food and water, even when that food and water were provided by feeding tube. This issue prompted intense discussion about exactly what should be done for the dying as far as food and fluids were concerned. While most agreed dying people should not have food *forced* upon them, there were differences of opinion regarding whether dying people should even be *offered* food and water.

Interestingly, in many institutions, CNAs who identified themselves as being from Jamaica reported that in their culture, the custom was to always give water to those who are dying. Food was not considered a necessity, but water, always. A number of Jamaican CNAs reported feeling especially good when they gave water to a resident shortly before the resident died.

In general, CNAs born outside the United States were more positive about feeding tubes and less likely to sanction the withholding or withdrawing of life-sustaining treatment. This is particularly noteworthy since many of the CNAs born outside the United States often mentioned that feeding tubes—as well as nursing homes—are rarely used in their countries. The idea that "we are here now and this is how things are done here" seemed to prevail.

C. DEGREE OF RELIGIOSITY

Prior to conducting this project, we had hypothesized that the CNAs' degree of religiosity would influence their feelings about their work in general, and about end-of-life issues in particular. Many CNAs are drawn from countries in which religion is highly regarded, and plays a part in the everyday lives of those who live there. Therefore, we assumed that religion—both religious affiliation and degree of religiosity—would play a role in how CNAs viewed many of the issues covered in this project.

CNAs were overwhelmingly drawn from a number of Christian denominations and were likely to describe themselves as very religious. And, as anticipated, the degree to which CNAs described themselves as religious was related to how they felt about certain end-of-life concerns. Of particular note were the issues related to resident autonomy, feeding, and comfort issues. For example, more religious CNAs tended to be in favor of using feeding tubes. Additionally, those who were more religious had greater difficulty with withholding or withdrawing life-sustaining treatment than were the less religious. Again, we could not be sure exactly why this was the case. However, we speculated that these were individuals who believed strongly that where there is life there is hope. Accordingly, they felt that the use of feeding tubes in many instances could prolong life for an extended period. As well, like many of their professional and lay counterparts, they may view withholding and withdrawing feeding tubes as "killing" a person, rather than seeing the underlying illness as the cause of death.

Also striking among the more religious CNAs was the tendency toward paternalism. Here, too, we could only guess why these two issues were associated. The possibility exists that this may be an extension of the high degree of paternalism found in many religions.

DIFFERENCES AMONG CNAS FROM RELIGIOUSLY-AFFILIATED NURSING HOMES

In addition to CNAs' individual characteristics and the role of these characteristics in how they view so many things, we also anticipated that their opinions on end-of-life care could be associated to some degree with the philosophy of their respective institutions about care of the dying and end-of-life decision-making. We were particularly interested in whether the culture of a particular facility might, in some way, influence how CNAs viewed many of the issues we focused on during the project.

Interestingly, findings about a number of issues varied considerably when viewed by individual nursing home. It is very difficult to even speculate why this occurred, but it may be related to the particular culture of a facility. However, with a few exceptions, given the relatively brief amount of time we spent in individual facilities, it was difficult in almost all situations for us to get a sense of the unique culture of each facility.

What we found, primarily, was that a facility's religious affiliation seemed to be associated with how CNAs felt about end-of-life issues. While we are not suggesting that a particular religious affiliation of a home will *cause* CNAs to feel a certain way, there were some interesting differences in viewpoints of CNAs from facilities under different religious auspices. In the Catholic facilities, for example, the CNAs were likely to feel that the spiritual needs of their residents were met. CNAs who worked in Jewish facilities were more likely to agree with the discontinuation of life-sustaining treatment, but were also more paternalistic. They were more likely to agree that patients preferred not to know they are dying, and that we should go along with families when they ask us not to tell a patient that he/she is dying. Subjects at Jewish facilities were also less likely to believe that it is possible to prevent dying residents from feeling much pain, and more likely to think that some of the treatments we give residents are too uncomfortable for them.

What is difficult to explain about the differences between CNAs in Jewish facilities and Catholic facilities is that all these CNAs are drawn from essentially the same pool. A lot of the issues they expressed feelings about are very personal and individual, with the exception of the CNAs in the Catholic facilities and their feelings about spiritual issues in their respective facilities. Clearly, further study is necessary to tease out these issues.

WHAT DOES THIS MEAN FOR THE CERTIFIED NURSING ASSISTANT?

CNAs need to be aware of the current thinking in health care on a number of issues. Clearly, one of these is respect for resident autonomy. As noted earlier, this may be difficult for CNAs drawn from ethnic backgrounds where this is not the norm. Two of the CNAs in one of the first educational sessions held during this project had an interaction we repeated regularly as the project progressed. While what they said focused only on feelings about nursing home use, the spirit of their words can be generalized to other issues, such as truth-telling and acknowledgment of resident autonomy.

In a discussion about placing elderly individuals in nursing homes, a nursing assistant from Trinidad stated, "In my country, we don't put people in nursing homes." Another nursing assistant responded, "Well, I'm from Ethiopia, and in my country, we don't put people in nursing homes either. However, I live here now, and I have two children in college. If I had to care for my parents at home, I would not be able to work, and I would not be able to pay for my children to go to college." While it may be difficult for some CNAs to accept certain facts of life in U.S. nursing homes, at least attempts should be made to raise their consciousness about the issues. They may not like to see a resident refuse a feeding tube, particularly when they have become attached to that resident. However, respecting a person's treatment wishes is mandated here, so we are obligated to go along with such requests, even when the result will be the death of the patient.

It must also be recognized that the work done by CNAs is truly emotionally draining, and that CNAs need emotional support. It is unrealistic for facilities to insist that CNAs remain emotionally uninvolved with their residents. It would clearly be more helpful to the nursing assistant and more beneficial to the resident if this fact is recognized and supported. In fact, some have found that CNAs' emotional attachment to residents enhances the care they provide at the end of their residents' lives (Wilson & Daley, 1998). Peer support can be used (Karioth, 1997) and the CNAs with whom we worked who supported and felt supported by their co-workers thought it was often very effective.

It would also be helpful to CNAs if nurses and social workers regularly acknowledged to CNAs that their work must be difficult, and how sad it must be for them when their residents die. The development and use of any mechanism that helps a nursing assistant to grieve and to carry these heavy emotional burdens (e.g., memorial services for residents) is a step in the right direction.

Interestingly, and sadly, while there is evidence that the gerontological community in general and nursing home administrations in particular are aware of the importance of nursing assistants, the CNAs themselves do not see that others view them so highly. Simply telling them we think they are valuable is clearly not the answer, and perhaps the nursing home industry must encourage other nursing home staff to recognize and appreciate the role played by CNAs. Many nursing home professionals make the erroneous assumption that their more advanced education makes them more knowledgeable about residents and resident care. To some degree, and on some level, this may be the case. However, it is the nursing assistant who spends, by far, the greatest amount of time with the resident. This fact alone gives her (or him) an incredible amount of knowledge of the resident's condition. It must be recognized in all nursing homes that optimum care can only be provided when all members of the caregiving team are respectful of and attentive to the importance of each member of the team.

REFERENCES

Cantor, M. H. (1983). Strain among caregivers. *The Gerontologist, 23*, 597–604.
Cantor, M. H., & Chichin, E. R. (1990). *Stress and strain among homecare workers of the frail elderly: Final report*. New York: Brookdale Research Institute on Aging, Third Age Center, Fordham University.
Foner, N. (1994). Nursing home aides: Saints or monsters? *The Gerontologist, 34*(2), 245–250.
Grau, L. A., Colombotos, J., & Gorman, S. (1992). Psychological morale and job satisfaction among home care worker who care for persons with AIDS. *Journal of Women and Health, 18*(1), 1–21.
Horowitz, A. (1985). Family caregiving to the frail elderly. In C. Eisdorfer (Ed.), *Annual Review of Gerontology and Geriatrics (Vol. 5)* (pp. 194–246). New York: Springer-Verlag.
Kane, R. A., & Caplan, A. L. (1991). *Everyday ethics*. New York: Springer.
Karioth, S. (1997). A loving good-bye. *Nursing Assistant Monthly, 4*(2), 2.
Libow, L. S., & Starer, P. (1989). Care of the nursing home patient. *New England Journal of Medicine, 321*(2), 93–96.

Looman, W. J., Noelker, L. S., Schur, D., Whitlatch, C. J., & Ejaz, F. (1997). Nursing assistants caring for dementia residents in nursing homes: The family's perspective on the high quality of care. *American Journal of Alzheimer's Care,* 221–226.

Wilson, S. A., & Daley, B. J. (1998). Attachment/detachment: Forces influencing care of the dying in long-term care. *Journal of Palliative Medicine, 1*(1), 21–34.

8

Respect for Autonomy: Opinions of CNAs

Respect for autonomy is the ethical principle that is regarded as the foundation of biomedical ethics in the United States. And, as was noted in the chapter on autonomy, it has been legislated in health care with the passage in 1991 of the federal Patient Self Determination Act. In conducting this project, we were interested in learning how much CNAs know about the concept of respect of autonomy and particularly how it is operationalized in health care settings. This was done by asking a series of questions about advance directives. These items clearly have right or wrong answers. We also wanted to know how they felt about specific issues associated with autonomy, and of course, these items had no right or wrong answers.

WHAT CNAs KNOW ABOUT AUTONOMY

CNAs regularly encounter many concrete manifestations of respect for autonomy, such as advance directives and truth-telling. Indeed, these are part of the daily work-life of the nursing assistant. We were particularly interested in knowing how knowledgeable CNAs are about some of these specific issues associated with autonomy. Thus, in addition to a number of items on the questionnaire, we also spent a fair amount of time in the educational sessions exploring these issues.

For better or worse, CNAs seemed to be as knowledgeable as the general public about these issues. That is to say, they did not know a great deal. However, we did not find this to be particularly surprising. While CNAs are employed in the health care field, it is clear that they are rarely exposed to the complex aspects associated with making treatment decisions for their residents. Often they do not even know who is involved in making treatment decisions, and rarely do they know if a decision reflects the resident's wishes. Thus, while they are the care givers who will actually be providing hands-on care while a treatment plan is being implemented, in most facilities they are left out of the decision-making loop.

Many report that they are often unaware of the existence of documents describing the treatment preferences of the residents for whom they care. As a rule, they have little or no contact with advance directives, and therefore are generally unaware of what authority they can confer, or the exact issues they can address. Repeatedly, they stated how much they would appreciate knowing in advance what a resident's wishes are with respect to end-of-life treatment. Then, if the time comes that a feeding tube is being considered, for example, and the resident left instructions that she would not want a feeding tube, the CNA is prepared for that eventuality.

Being out of the decision-making loop has even more complex implications in New York State. In New York, when a patient cannot make his treatment preferences known and there are no advance directives, there must be "clear and convincing evidence" of wishes to limit life-sustaining treatment. This evidence is generally in the form of written or oral statements that people may have made regarding their feelings about a particular treatment in a particular instance. However, CNAs are not usually privy to discussions with families or friends in which the resident's treatment preferences may have been outlined. As a result, they generally have absolutely no idea how a decision may have been made to limit treatment, and may assume it is only because the family wanted this course of action, and not because the resident may have wanted it and the family is acting in his or her behalf.

Interestingly, the CNAs from New York State were more knowledgeable about the specifics of advance directives than were the CNAs from New Jersey. Again, we can only speculate why this occurs. We suspect this may be a function of the particularly stringent laws with respect to treatment decision-making in New York (i.e., the fact that an advance directive or clear and convincing evidence of an individual's desire to limit life-sustaining treatment is necessary when making treatment decisions for persons without decision-making capacity). It may be that in New Jersey, it is a little easier to limit some treatments at the end of life. Therefore, less attention is paid to these issues in educational sessions with nursing assistants.

ATTITUDES ABOUT ETHICAL ISSUES AND END-OF-LIFE DECISION-MAKING

While respect for autonomy is the law, we were aware that feelings about this ethical principle may vary greatly from individual to individual. This was the case with the CNAs in this project as well. Not surprisingly, we found CNAs with whom we worked viewing the subject from different perspectives. Issues associated with autonomy often encouraged heated debates in the educational sessions.

Again, we could only speculate why an individual nursing assistant felt the way she (or he) did about respect for autonomy. One possible factor could be socioeconomic status. Almost all CNAs are drawn from lower income and lower educational levels. This has limited their ability to make any choices in life; rather, they simply are forced to take what life gives them. The concept of autonomy, of making a free choice, may be totally alien to them.

Another factor that may influence how CNAs feel is their cultural backgrounds. Many CNAs are from countries where the idea of autonomy—particularly individual patient autonomy—is completely foreign. In the most extreme, in many countries, physicians alone make health care decisions for patients. In less extreme cases, the family is the decision-maker, often completely without the involvement of the patient. (See for example, Surbone, 1992.)

Yet another issue that may be associated with why CNAs feel the way they do about autonomy is the influence of the professionals with whom they work. Although they are obliged by law to respect patients' wishes with respect to treatment, many health care professionals have great difficulty doing so, particularly when the professional believes he or she knows what is best for the resident. This may be easily communicated to the nursing assistants, who then may begin to feel the same way.

The CNAs' knowledge base regarding ethical issues can obviously be increased. Attitudes, on the other hand, are often deeply ingrained and difficult to alter. While participating in this project may not have changed the attitudes of the CNAs about these issues, it may have raised their consciousness about them. In some way, it may make CNAs more accepting of residents' choices, even when those choices may conflict with what they might want for the resident, or what they would want for themselves. Several CNAs told us that in the past, they generally accepted feeding tubes as the norm. Now, they said, when they see a resident with a feeding tube, they wonder what the resident's wishes were with respect to artificial nutrition and hydration, and how the decision to insert the tube was made.

The CNAs participating in this project made it very clear that they felt strongly that residents have the right to make their own decisions about treatment. On both the pre and posttest questionnaires, as well as in the education sessions, very high proportions of CNAs stated that residents have the right to refuse treatments, even if those treatments are necessary to prolong their lives. In the ensuing discussions, however, CNAs spent a great deal of time discussing the difficulties associated with actually implementing these requests to limit treatment. While they believe strongly that residents have these rights, the CNAs are often distressed because they generally become very attached to their residents, and are greatly saddened by the inevitable outcome (i.e., the death of a resident) when life-sustaining treatment is limited.

The subject of truth-telling was also quite provocative. CNAs felt strongly that they should protect residents from information that might be distressing to them (e.g., the death of an adult child, a serious illness, etc.), and the CNAs often came across to us as being quite paternalistic. Where issues of truth-telling were concerned, large proportions of CNAs stated they felt we should respect the requests of families not to reveal information that they felt might be upsetting to the resident, even though respect for autonomy mandates that residents have a right to the information.

There was also discussion of a person's right to know his or her diagnosis, particularly if that diagnosis involved a terminal illness. CNAs had strong feelings about revealing terminal diagnoses in general, and spent a great deal of discussion time on this topic. Interestingly, this issue tended to be personalized by the CNAs. In the discussion sessions, many CNAs prefaced their opinions with the phrase, "If it were me. . . . " Generally, in every nursing home educational session, there were CNAs who said they would never want to know if they had a terminal diagnosis. Often, however, they would say they would like to know the illness was very serious, but they would not like to know an exact prognosis. Those who stated they would like to know if their condition was terminal talked about the need to make arrangements for children, to right old wrongs, or to generally just "set their houses in order."

As far as treatment decision-making was concerned, CNAs generally felt residents should be able to refuse life-sustaining treatment, and should not have such treatments "forced" upon them against their will. When it came to artificial nutrition, however, there was clearly a great deal of ambivalence.

Given our interest in and concern about the appropriate use of comfort care in nursing homes, we generally favor limiting the use of artificial nutrition and hydration at the very end of life. Prior to conducting the study, we had hypothesized that many CNAs would also find the use of feeding tubes and IVs in dying patients to be burdensome forms of treatment. Surprisingly, however, many of the CNAs found feeding tubes to be highly acceptable. In fact, it was obvious to us that tubes are perceived as the norm when it came to long term care of residents. Of note, however, was what CNAs said when we asked them what they would want for themselves. In discussions in the educational sessions about whether they would like feeding tubes for themselves were they in the conditions that many of their residents manifested, relatively few CNAs answered in the affirmative. In fact, in discussing feeding tubes in general, many CNAs opined that they would accept tubes for themselves only for a very limited time period, if at all.

Also of note, as mentioned in the chapter on CNAs and how they see themselves, were the differences in views on autonomy between CNAs who were U.S.-born and those who were born in the Caribbean. CNAs born in the United States were more likely to be in favor of respecting resident autonomy than were those from the Caribbean. Caribbean-born CNAs were also more paternalistic, agreeing that we should go along with families when they ask us not to tell a patient that he/she is dying.

WHAT DOES THIS MEAN FOR THE CNA?

Obviously, as stated at the beginning of this chapter, we felt that we would be able, through this program, to increase the knowledge base of CNAs about ethical issues. We were also doubtful that we would be able to change their attitudes. At the conclusion of the project, it was clear that this supposition was correct. But, again as noted earlier, we did seem to raise consciousness about many of these issues.

Nursing assistants ought to have a working knowledge of advance directives: what they are, and what they are not. They should also be aware of who among the residents they care for has an advance directive of any sort. This gives the CNA a better picture of the resident overall, and prepares the CNA for the eventuality that there may be a time when the use of life-sustaining treatments may be limited, if that is the resident's previously-stated wish.

CNAs also need to understand that it is acceptable for them to have their own opinions about life-sustaining treatment, and that they have every right to make health care decisions for themselves. What they do not have, and what their professional counterparts do not have, is the right to make decisions for others. It may be very difficult to accept a resident's choice to limit life-sustaining treatment. But, it is the resident's choice. That cannot be overemphasized.

As noted in the previous chapter, CNAs need a clear understanding of the ethical principle of respect for autonomy, both in everyday decisions as well as end-of-life treatment decisions for nursing home residents. In order to provide the best possible resident care, it is imperative that we recognize that CNAs will very likely have difficulty respecting the autonomy of residents, for all the reasons stated above. It will be particularly difficult for them when the outcome of respecting what the resident would want for himself or herself will result in the death of the resident. And it will be even more distressing when the CNA has grown very close to the resident. The other thing that we in nursing homes must continue to do is to educate CNAs about respecting autonomy and their role in this process, and to support them as they do so.

REFERENCES

Surbone, A. (1992). Letter from Italy: Truth-telling to the patient. *Journal of the American Medical Association, 268*(13), 1661–1662.

9

Comfort Care and the CNA

The focus of all care in nursing homes should be on the comfort of the resident and attention to comfort should be implicit in all we do in the health care setting. Unfortunately, however, while comfort care should always be prioritized, it often falls by the wayside in an age where technological medical care reigns supreme. For too long now, comfort care has been awarded second-class status. A main goal of this project was to make CNAs realize that there is something wrong with this picture, and that they have an important role in righting this wrong.

We spent a great deal of discussion time talking about just what constitutes comfort care, and perhaps most important, the role that CNAs have in providing it. Under the umbrella term "comfort care," we focused on the appropriate use of treatments such as artificial nutrition and hydration, antibiotics for infection, and amputation of limbs for gangrene. We discussed pain and symptom control, and stressed the many things that CNAs could do to make residents more comfortable, particularly in the case of residents who were refusing life-sustaining treatment. And finally, we asked CNAs what they saw as barriers to good care.

REFUSAL OF LIFE-SUSTAINING TREATMENT AND CARE OF THE DYING

As noted above, comfort care should be provided throughout an individual's nursing home stay. However, it becomes paramount as death becomes more imminent. In a number of cases, particularly when a nursing home resident has exercised the right to autonomy by asking that life-sustaining treatment be limited, the use of aggressive comfort care is imperative.

The refusal of life-sustaining treatment by a nursing home resident generally results in the start of the process of dying and the subsequent death of the resident. We anticipated that CNAs might have a problem with the idea that residents legally and ethically are permitted to refuse treatment. While this did turn out to be the case in many instances, it was generally the potential death of the resident that was the issue. As noted elsewhere, CNAs generally felt residents should be able to refuse life-sustaining treatment. They were almost unanimous is stating that residents should never have such treatments "forced" upon them against their will. However, when it came to the use of artificial nutrition and hydration, there were clearly mixed feelings.

As noted elsewhere, many of the CNAs found feeding tubes to be so acceptable that they were seen as the norm when it came to long term care of residents. Thus, asking them to think about the appropriate use of artificial nutrition and hydration for their residents was highly provocative. A substantial amount of time was spent in the educational sessions discussing feelings about feeding tubes, and asking CNAs to question the extent to which they should be used.

We discussed the numerous meanings associated with food in every culture. Information contained in the excellent article by Jacqueline Slomka (1995), "What Do Apple Pie and Motherhood Have to Do with Feeding Tubes and Caring for the Patient?" was shared with the CNAs and served as a springboard for further discussion. Slomka's provocative piece focuses on all the emotional issues associated with food, and the difficulties health care professionals (and, as we are seeing, their paraprofessional counterparts) have when we equate the medical procedure of tube feeding with all the cultural and nurturant characteristics associated with food. "What do you think?" we asked. "When we use a feeding tube, are we talking about food, or medical treatment?" Like most of the lay public and a large number of their professional counterparts, CNAs saw these concepts as blurred, although many in health care agree feeding tubes constitute medical treatment. We shared with the CNAs Slomka's (1995) suggestion that using the term "forced feeding" instead of "tube feeding" might encourage people to think differently.

PAIN AND SYMPTOM CONTROL

Of concern to the CNAs, as well as to health care professionals and the lay public, is the belief that patients who do not receive artificial nutrition and hydration will suffer terribly because they are "starving to death." A great deal of time was spent in the educational sessions discussing what actually happens when this choice is made and implemented, focusing on the fact that when a person is taking no nourishment and we do not administer artificial fluids death results from dehydration.

The feelings that are experienced by an individual who opts not to have artificial nutrition and hydration are not what we feel when we skip a meal. We noted that considerable emphasis is placed on terminal dehydration in the literature. This literature attests to the fact that dying without artificial nutrition and hydration is strongly believed by many to be far more comfortable than dying artificially hydrated (Ahronheim, 1996; Billings, 1985; Brody, Campbell, Faber-Langendoen, & Ogle, 1997; McCann, Hall, & Growth-Junker, 1994; Printz, 1992; Sullivan, 1993; Zerwekh, 1983, 1997). Not using artificial hydration at the end of life reduces the possibility of fluid overload. It minimizes the production of urine, decreasing the need to disturb the patient. It lessens respiratory secretions, thereby reducing if not eliminating the need for suctioning. As well, it "de-medicalizes" the environment and the dying process. It is nature's way of dying, the way people have died for centuries and still die today in many situations.

We stressed to the CNAs that terminal dehydration leads to chemical changes in the body that tend to have a sedating effect. Also emphasized was the work of McCann and his colleagues (1994). In a study conducted with dying patients who were able to communicate how they felt (as opposed to most dying nursing home residents who, because of dementia, do not have that capability), McCann et al. (1994) found no complaints of hunger. Rather, the most frequently-occurring complaint was of dry mouth. This symptom was easily relieved by small sips of water and good mouth care. Particularly noteworthy is that, assuming adequate pain control, meticulous mouth care may be the most important component of good comfort care, and clearly is something that falls to the nursing assistant!

There was considerable discussion about giving pain medication to relieve suffering. As noted in the "Results" chapter, only about half the CNAs felt it is acceptable to give pain medication to relieve suffering, if so doing may make the resident die sooner. Responses to this item served as a springboard for a discussion of the principle of double effect. This concept states that if the primary goal of an act is good, and there is a secondary negative result, then the act is acceptable, based on its primary goal (Beauchamp & Childress, 1989).

Another related issue centers on the use of morphine in patients with end-stage dementia who are close to death and are manifesting some signs of discomfort (e.g., moaning or rapid breathing). We regularly use small doses (2 to 4 mg. subcutaneously every four to six hours) for dying dementia patients whom we suspect are uncomfortable but, as a result of their illness, are unable to express how they feel. As with our experience with staff members caring for nearly 300 residents referred to The Jewish Home's ethics consult team, we found a good deal of variation in the attitudes toward the use of morphine expressed by CNAs. We have encountered many nurses and physicians who dislike using morphine in cases where they do not have a patient who is complaining of severe pain, despite the insignificant size of the dose, and the fact that it is the drug of choice for pain and terminal dyspnea (Enck, 1994). This phenomenon is one we have not been able to explain, although we have speculated that perhaps the use of morphine in these cases is perceived by some as tantamount to euthanasia. Hopefully, as initiatives focusing on pain management grow across the country, professionals and paraprofessionals in health care settings will begin to have more positive feelings toward the use of this most useful intervention.

THE USE OF BURDENSOME TREATMENTS

The issue of using burdensome treatments on nursing home residents was the focus of part of the educational sessions. As noted earlier, prior to conducting the study, we had hypothesized that many CNAs would find the use of artificial nutrition and hydration to be burdensome for the resident. Tube feedings require insertion of a tube into the abdomen or through the nose. Artificial hydration necessitates venipuncture, a procedure that often must be repeated on a frail elderly individual with poor venous access. In addition, while increasing numbers of facilities are doing so, many nursing homes do not provide artificial hydration, and residents who require it are hospitalized. Nonetheless, CNAs found artificial nutrition and hydration to be the norm, and tended to be quite accepting of these procedures. So, although we often saw the use of tube feedings and intravenous therapy to be burdensome, most CNAs did not.

With respect to other treatments, CNAs were somewhat split in their feelings about whether some of the treatments we give to residents are too uncomfortable. Those CNAs who did feel that residents received burdensome treatments were more likely to cite treatments that they themselves were required to administer. One of the more frequently mentioned uncomfortable treatments was the application of splints to contracted limbs. CNAs reported that this caused great pain to residents, and given a choice, they would much prefer not using splints, and perhaps bathing the limb in warm water to make it more pliable.

Another task which they had difficulty performing was getting a resident out of bed when they felt the resident was exceedingly weak, or if the resident had a bedsore. In these cases, the CNAs would have much preferred to keep the resident in bed, and position her from side to side every two hours. When they asked the nurses about this, however, the nurses suggested that they were simply lazy, and anyway, "the State" says the residents must be taken out of bed every day.

BARRIERS TO GOOD CARE

As noted earlier, when asked what CNAs saw as barriers to good care, the two most prominent areas were insufficient staff and fear of being sued. The fact that not enough staff was cited as a problem was not surprising; this is a chronic complaint in health care facilities, and clearly may have some legitimacy. Given the multitude of tasks associated with caring for just one frail elderly individual, and multiplying that by eight or ten or more, the amount of work assigned to CNAs can be overwhelming.

The degree to which CNAs expressed concern about fear of lawsuits, however, was unanticipated, especially since it was explained to the CNAs during the data collection period that we were not asking if they were concerned about lawsuits directed toward them specifically, but rather lawsuits in which the facility would be sued.

In one facility, the CNAs were particularly concerned about lawsuits. This was in a nursing home that regularly sent its CNAs to outside inservices, and several of them had attended a program on bedsores. In the course of the program, the speaker stressed that nursing homes can be sued when residents develop bedsores. This information was disseminated to most of the other CNAs in the facility, resulting in a heightened awareness of the possibility of lawsuits.

WHAT DOES ALL THIS MEAN FOR THE NURSING ASSISTANT?

As noted above, assuming adequate pain and symptom management, the majority of comfort care is provided by nursing assistants. This fact cannot be stressed too highly. And, while CNAs cannot administer medication, they should be aware that medication is available to treat most symptoms evident at the end of life.

Also worthy of emphasis is the role of nursing assistants in symptom observation. The long term care nurse, no matter how conscientious and caring, cannot observe changes in symptoms in all her residents with any degree of frequency. CNAs, on the other hand, spend an enormous amount of time with residents, and clearly know them best. Thus, it falls to the nursing assistant to note and report to the nurse any symptoms of discomfort noted in the resident. Accordingly, CNAs need to be educated as to what symptoms are noteworthy and should be reported.

Given CNAs' general acceptance of feeding tubes and intravenous therapy as the norm in long term care, it may be difficult to dispel this notion. The CNAs in our project may have begun to view forgoing life-sustaining treatment as less appalling than before. However, there were still a significant number who remained distressed at the prospect. Changing this mind-set will most likely take some time and effort.

It is clear that changing the mind-set regarding comfort care in nursing homes must be geared to more than just CNAs. For it to be effective, all levels of staff must be conversant with the principles of good comfort care. This is obviously a challenge, although not necessarily an insurmountable one.

REFERENCES

Ahronheim, J. (1996). Nutrition and hydration in the terminal patient. *Clinics in Geriatric Medicine, 12*(2), 379–391.

Beauchamp, T. L., & Childress, J. F. (1989). *Principles of medical ethics* (3rd ed.). New York: Oxford University Press.

Billings, J. A. (1985). Comfort measures for the terminally ill: Is dehydration painful? *Journal of the American Geriatrics Society, 33*(11), 808–810.

Brody, H., Campbell, M. L., Faber-Langendoen, K., & Ogle, K. S. (1997). Withdrawing intensive life-sustaining treatment: Recommendations for compassionate clinical management. *New England Journal of Medicine, 336*(9), 652–657.

Enck, R. E. (1994). *Medical care of the terminally ill.* Baltimore, MD: Johns Hopkins University Press.

McCann, R. M., Hall, W. J., & Groth-Juncker, A. (1994). Comfort care for terminally ill patients: The appropriate use of nutrition and hydration. *Journal of the American Medical Association, 272*(16), 1263–1266.

Printz, L. A. (1992). Terminal dehydration: A compassionate treatment. *Archives of Internal Medicine, 152*, 697–700.

Slomka, J. (1995). What do apple pie and motherhood have to do with feeding tubes and caring for the patient? *Archives of Internal Medicine, 155*(12), 1258–1263.

Sullivan, R. J. (1993). Accepting death without artificial nutrition or hydration. *Journal of General Internal Medicine, 8*, 220–224.

Zerwekh, J. V. (1983, January). The dehydration question. *Nursing, 83*, 47–51.

Zerwekh, J. V. (1997). Do dying patients really need IV fluids? *American Journal of Nursing, 97*(3), 26–30.

10

CNAs' Evaluations of the Educational Ethics Program

We were very interested in learning how the CNAs felt about this program, and their participation in it. Accordingly, following the intervention sessions, subjects in the experimental group were asked to complete a short evaluation form assessing the ethics education program. The form contained ten close-ended questions. Subjects were asked to indicate on a Likert scale ranging from (1) "not at all" to (5) "very much" how they felt about each of the questions. Higher scores indicated a more positive assessment of the program (see TABLE 10.1 for a summary of subjects' responses). The questionnaire also contained five open-ended questions in which subjects were asked to describe in more detail their feelings about the program. Examples of these questions included: "What did you like most about the sessions?" "What did you like least about the sessions?" and "Are there any topics that you think we should have discussed that were not discussed at all or were not discussed in enough detail?" (See Appendix B for a copy of the entire Ethics Education Evaluation Form).

As can be seen from subjects' responses to both the open-ended (see below) and close-ended questions (see TABLE 10.1), CNAs had very positive feelings about participating in the program. CNAs generally found the topics interesting, relevant to their work, and helpful to themselves and their coworkers. Additionally, participants enjoyed the opportunity to express their own views about the issues as well as to benefit from listening to the thoughts and feelings of other CNAs. While CNAs often interact in their units, they do not usually have the opportunity to discuss end-of-life issues about residents with each other or other staff members. As has been discussed throughout this book, CNAs are typically left out of discussions concerning resident care planning and are often not even aware of key issues affecting the individuals for whom they provide care. A number of CNAs stated that these sessions gave them a better understanding of the factors involved in end-of-life decision-making and care.

In the open-ended questions subjects often mentioned how important it is for them to learn about end-of-life issues and how to better care for dying residents. CNAs found these issues relevant not only to their professional lives but to their personal lives as well. A number of CNAs stated that they were experiencing many of the same concerns with their own family members as were addressed during the educational sessions (e.g., completing advance directives, making a decision about a feeding tube placement, medication choices,

TABLE 10.1   CNAs Evaluation of the Ethics Education Program

Question	Not at all		Somewhat		Very much	Mean Score
	1	2	3	4	5	
Do you feel that you personally needed these sessions?	4.8%	1.6%	25.4%	15.5%	52.8%	4.10
Do you feel that other nursing assistants in the group needed the sessions?	2.0%	2.8%	29.0%	15.5%	50.8%	4.10
Do you think the sessions were interesting?	0.4%	0.4%	7.9%	6.7%	84.5%	4.75
Do you feel that you learned anything new in the sessions?	0.8%	2.0%	20.6%	7.5%	69.0%	4.42
Did you feel that you could speak openly about your feelings towards the different topics discussed during the sessions?	0.8%	0.8%	14.2%	10.7%	73.4%	4.55
Do you think that participating in these sessions will help you in your job?	2.8%	0.8%	20.1%	17.7%	58.6%	4.29
Would you recommend this ethics education program to other nursing assistants?	0.4%	0.4%	10.4%	13.6%	75.2%	4.63
Would you want to go to more ethics sessions like this one in the future?	2.8%	2.0%	16.1%	12.4%	66.7%	4.38
Was it helpful to have the opportunity to discuss these issues with other nursing assistants?	0.4%	1.2%	17.9%	12.6%	67.9%	4.46
Did you like hearing what other nursing assistants had to say about these issues?	0.4%	1.2%	10.2%	32.9%	55.3%	4.42

etc.). They found it helpful to hear different points of view as well as learn more about their options.

One of the factors of the program that CNAs especially appreciated and commented on was that the program made them feel that their opinions are important and the work they do is valuable. This is an important aspect of the program considering the crucial work that CNAs do within the nursing home along with the finding that they often feel their opinions are not respected by the people they work with (see chapter 7).

Negative comments were very few and far between. The main criticism of the program was that it was too short and too few CNAs attended. This was mentioned by several of the CNAs. The most requested additional program was a session dealing with death and care of the dying patient, and comments about care of the dying were the second most frequently mentioned issue in the evaluations.

A selection of some of the positive comments follows:

It helped me to understand about the dying patient better, and hear different things about other nursing homes.

The sessions gave me new ideas of how to relate to a patient who is dying and to the caregivers.

We need any inservices that will teach us to care more for the residents . . . the most important inservice program we need is how to deal with patients dying after getting close to them.

There was not enough time to bring out the many things I want to know about the ways of dealing with death and dying.

Every nursing assistant should be involved in these sessions. Mainly because there will come a time in life they will need these sessions very much. This session pretty much said a lot—dealing with death of the elderly and family members. It helps you understand so much!

I would like to learn more about how to deal with the family of a dying patient and how to deal with a terminal patient.

I like the fact that we were allowed to voice our opinions about the topics and most of all that you listened. This session came right on time because I'm going through this myself with my aunt. I'm her proxy and she's in a nursing home. I wish these sessions were longer. Maybe it would be easier for me to make these decisions for my aunt. These sessions have been a godsend.

I feel this was a very informative and open-minded session. I found it to be very enlightening and stimulating just to know how others feel. I do not feel that death is a terrible thing but can be a beautiful and peaceful phase of life.

The remaining comments focused on appreciation for the program in general, and gratitude for feeling respected in particular:

Such sessions should be held every six months.

I enjoyed all five sessions. It was a great idea to bring this program to our nursing home.

I enjoyed all the topics that were discussed. It helped me to understand the needs of the residents and their rights. I also told my coworkers about it.

I think that the nurses need to learn to respect our views. We know more about the patient than anyone else.

I learned more about issues in resident care facilities which I didn't know much about hitherto. I got enough explanations to either maintain, change, or disregard most of my opinions. At some point I realized that most of my colleagues had very strong opinions about certain issues, and no matter what, it was hard to convince them. But, in my opinion, this program basically covered almost all the essential topics that nursing assistants need to keep up with.

It was a pleasure to come to these sessions because I learned a lot.

I think it would be valuable to have this type of program throughout the year.

This was a well-run program (and) I'd like to have more programs like this.

This class was great!

I think every nursing home should have an ethics program.

I enjoyed the sessions and I learned a lot.

(What I liked least about the sessions was that) they took me away from my work BUT I DID NOT MIND (sic).

(What I liked most about the sessions was the) freedom to express my opinions and they were respected. There wasn't anything I disliked about the sessions. The person who was in charge was very pleasant and easy-going and appeared to care deeply about our opinions and thoughts. It was rather pleasant being a part of these sessions.

It was a pleasure being in this program.

(I liked these sessions because) you listened to us and you think our job is important too!

(I liked these sessions because) you are able to state your opinions and have someone there to listen to you. It was a great program—very helpful and meaningful.

(I liked these sessions because) it gave me a chance to express myself and helped me understand more about life. I wish we could get together real soon—I enjoyed it very much.

I really enjoyed every minute of this program and I thank you for making me a part of it.

I felt good after I left each session and I looked forward to the next one.

I liked that we all had different opinions and we heard those different opinions that help us look at things in a different way.

I like speaking openly about different things. I really enjoyed this program because later in the future we may have to really think about these things.

I have no complaints about this program—I just hope to have more like this in the future.

I really enjoyed this inservice, I found it to be very interesting and educational. I also learned the feelings of my coworkers. Please come again!

I would like to have more inservices where we could give our opinions. We are not asked often and I think at times what we have to say could be very important.

I think this program was very meaningful to us. And it was well appreciated.

I appreciated being part of this program. I feel that talking about these issues informally helped to clarify my own feelings. Thank you *very* much!

This inservice helped me personally look at the way I really felt about these issues—which was comforting even to myself.

These sessions made me feel like my opinion and job is important. Keep up the good work. I think you are making CNAs feel like we are important.

I really liked that our opinions were respected and that someone listened to us.

I really liked that we had a chance to speak to someone who respects us and cares about our feelings.

While we felt that this was a useful and beneficial program for nursing assistants, we were particularly pleased that CNAs found it useful as well. The evaluations are clearly highly positive, and should encourage other facilities to focus on the issues associated with CNAs and ethics at the end of life in the nursing home, in addition to related topics suggested by the CNAs.

11

The Certified Nursing Assistant Support Group Program

In addition to the primary study using an educational intervention, we conducted a support group program with a smaller sample of CNAs. While the main focus of the larger study was to educate CNAs about end-of-life ethics, the primary objective of the support program was to provide CNAs with a reassuring environment in which they could discuss their experiences and feelings caring for dying residents. Again special attention was focused on the experience of caring for residents who died after refusing life-sustaining treatment.

There has been growing recognition over the last many years concerning the emotional and psychological needs of health care workers caring for dying patients. A number of articles have been written by nurses discussing the feelings of grief and distress that they themselves have experienced on the job over the loss of a patient (Sheard, 1984; Sonstegard, Hansen, Zillman, & Johnson, 1976). In general, these papers have been written in response to an underlying belief that traditional nursing education has emphasized the maintenance of control and composure over one's feelings in the heath care setting, and has not legitimized the expression of grief over the loss of a patient. While health care workers often experience multiple losses in their profession they usually do not receive the support that is available to family and friends mourning a death (Lev, 1989). Dealing with one's grief however may be necessary for nursing staff to effectively care for dying patients on an ongoing basis (Sonstegard et al., 1976).

While much of the literature has focused on the needs and experiences of hospice and acute care staff, there is evidence that staff within the long term care setting also experience feelings of grief. Lerea and LiMauro (1982) examined the grief responses of nurses and nursing assistants working in hospitals and nursing homes. Sixty-three percent of the nursing home nurses and nursing assistants reported feelings of grief in response to a patient's "physical or emotional experience." Additionally, 38 percent of staff reported symptoms of grief persisting for more than a month. While the experience of grief was found to be significantly more prevalent among hospital staff (98%), the large number of nursing home workers who reported grief responses should not be ignored. Lereo and LiMauro (1982) speculated that nursing home staff may experience less grief due to the expected death of elderly residents. These residents often decline over years due to chronic illness, and death may be seen as an end to this suffering. In comparison, hospital patients are often younger and death may be unexpected.

In recent years, however, the care of dying elderly nursing home residents has become more complex. Since the passage of the federal Patient Self Determination Act (1991), health care providers and health care institutions are mandated to give priority to the patient's treatment preferences, even when the patient chooses to limit the use of life-sustaining treatment. Patients and residents may decide that they prefer to focus on the benefits of comfort care rather than curative treatment if there is little or no chance of recovery and they are unsatisfied with the quality of life that will likely follow (e.g., fed by feeding tube, dementia, pain, etc.). Thus, in addition to the difficulty of losing a resident that one has cared for, often for long periods of time, staff must accept some residents' choices not to continue life-sustaining treatment, even when the continuation of treatment could theoretically prolong a resident's life for years (e.g., the insertion of a feeding tube). This situation may be especially difficult for nursing assistants who provide the day-to-day care of residents but are typically not included in discussions of treatment. Nursing assistants may be informed that aggressive medical treatment will no longer be provided to a resident, but not necessarily how this decision was made or whether it is in accordance with the resident's wishes. Moreover, after the decision to end aggressive treatment has been made, it is the nursing assistant who continues to provide care for the resident throughout the dying process.

Administrative staff in nursing homes are often unaware of the emotional needs of their nurses and nursing assistants who care for the dying. A recent study by Wilson and Daley (1998) found that staff at all levels of the nursing home hierarchy, including housekeeping, nursing assistants, nurses, and administrators develop feelings of attachment to residents and experience sadness when a resident dies. Additionally, administrators were aware that strong attachments develop between staff and residents. However, they were unaware of the intensity of the loss experienced by staff at the death of a resident. Similar results were found by Robbins, Lloyd, Carpenter, and Bender (1992). Management and supervisory staff in a residential home for the elderly were unaware of the level of anxiety that their nursing assistants experienced in relation to care of the dying. In our experience, it is rare to come across a nursing home that provides ongoing supportive programs to staff caring for dying residents.

The purpose of the present support program study was twofold. First, it explored CNAs' feelings, experiences, and needs when caring for the dying. Special attention was focused on the care of residents who have opted not to continue life-sustaining treatment. Secondly, the efficacy of this type of support program for CNAs was examined.

METHODS

This project took place at two large urban nursing homes that had not been part of the larger study. Thirty-five CNAs in groups of four to eight participated in five one-hour discussion sessions. Participants were selected by nursing management and all had cared for residents who died after life-sustaining treatment was refused. All participating CNAs were from the day and evening shifts.

The group sessions were facilitated by one of the Principal Investigators and/or the Project Director. The initial group session was joined by Kenneth Doka, PhD, a gerontologist and certified death education counselor, who served as a consultant on the project.

In the first session, an overview of the program was provided to the CNAs explaining the reason and rationale for the program. The CNAs were informed that the program was part of a larger project designed to provide ethics education and support to CNAs working in long term care facilities. They were also told that this part of the project would focus less on the educational component and more on their thoughts and feelings about caring for dying residents. The CNAs were told that all of their individual comments would remain confidential.

The discussions in the group sessions were loosely guided by the facilitators. The CNAs were encouraged to talk about their experiences caring for dying residents. In particular they were asked to discuss: the type of support they receive when caring for dying residents, their relationships with residents, the most difficult aspects of their jobs, what they find helps them cope when caring for dying residents, and those things they feel would be beneficial when working with the dying.

To facilitate discussion, CNAs were given a short questionnaire (see TABLE 11.1 for all of the items on the questionnaire) to complete during the first or second session. The first half of the questionnaire contained seven statements about care of the dying. CNAs were asked to indicate on a five-point scale how strongly they agreed or disagreed with each of the statements. In the second section of the questionnaire, CNAs were presented

TABLE 11.1   Results of the Staff Questionnaire: Part 1

	% of Subjects who Responded:					
Question	Strongly Agree	Agree	Don't Know	Disagree	Strongly Disagree	Mean
1. I think that caring for a person who is dying is always emotionally draining.	22%	52%	0%	15%	11%	2.41
2. Caring for a person who is dying can be a very rewarding experience.	19%	59%	0%	22%	0%	2.26
3. Caring for people who are dying can be a very rewarding experience, even if they are dying because they refused to have a feeding tube.	18%	32%	11%	39%	0%	2.71
4. It is more difficult to care for a person who is dying because they refused to have a feeding tube than it is to care for a person who is dying from a disease they have no control over.	22%	26%	4%	44%	4%	2.82
5. People who do not want life-sustaining treatment (for example, a feeding tube) should not be admitted to a nursing home.	0%	0%	4%	74%	22%	4.19
6. If I had a choice, I would rather NOT be assigned to a person who is dying from a disease they have no control over.	4%	4%	0%	78%	15%	3.96
7. If a resident chooses to have a treatment discontinued and will die as a result, I would respect that decision and willingly care for the resident during the dying process.	44%	44%	4%	4%	4%	1.78

Note: Lower mean score indicates greater agreement (1 = Strongly Agree; 5 = Strongly Disagree).

TABLE 11.1   Results of the Staff Questionnaire: Part 2

Question	% of Subjects who Responded:				
	Always	Sometimes	Rarely	Never	Mean
1. I feel helpless.	27%	54%	12%	8%	2.00
2. I feel sad.	57%	38%	0%	0%	1.37
3. I feel as if I have no control over what is happening.	27%	55%	9%	9%	2.00
4. I feel as if I'm not doing my job well enough.	8%	13%	21%	58%	3.29
5. I feel stressed.	13%	79%	4%	4%	2.00
6. I feel there is no one I can talk to about what is happening.	4%	44%	28%	24%	2.72

Note: A lower mean score indicates the event is more likely to happen (1 = Always; 4 = Never).

with a list of six statements describing different feelings (e.g., "I feel sad," "I feel stressed," "I feel I have no one to talk to"). They were asked to indicate on a 4-point scale ranging from "never" to "always" how often they experience each of the feelings when caring for dying residents (see TABLE 11.1 for the items on the questionnaire).

At the end of the last session the CNAs were asked to evaluate the program by completing a second short questionnaire (see TABLE 11.2 for a copy of the evaluation questionnaire).

RESULTS

RESPONSES TO STAFF QUESTIONNAIRE

The results of the Staff Questionnaire are presented in TABLE 11.1. As can be seen the majority of CNAs "agreed" (52%) or "strongly agreed" (22%) that caring for a dying person is always emotionally draining. Additionally, many CNAs often reported feelings of distress when working with the dying. Fifty-four percent of subjects stated they "sometimes" feel helpless when caring for the dying, and as many as 27% said they "always" feel this way. Only 8% reported never feeling helpless in these situations. Moreover, all CNAs stated they "sometimes" (38%) or "always" (62%) feel sad when caring for the dying.

In response to whether they experience stress when caring for dying residents, 92% of the subjects said they felt stressed at least some of the time. During discussion it was apparent that much of the stress results from CNAs' intensive workload. Subjects felt they could not spend as much time with each resident, particularly dying residents, as they or the residents would like due to the competing needs of others under their care. Subjects were split concerning whether they felt there is no one they can talk to when caring for dying residents. Almost half responded "sometimes" (44%) or "always" (4%) to this question.

Many subjects reported feeling as if they had no control over what is happening when they work with the dying (27% "always" and 55% "sometimes"). This, however, appeared to be an adaptive response for many CNAs. CNAs said they know are doing their best for the resident and they accept their limitations. They know that it is often not within their

TABLE 11.2   CNAs' Evaluation of the Support Program

Questions	Not at all		Somewhat		Very much	Mean Score
	1	2	3	4	5	
Do you feel that you personally needed these sessions?	0%	0%	30%	20%	50%	4.20
Do you feel that other nursing assistants in the group needed the sessions?	0%	0%	50%	10%	40%	3.90
Do you think the sessions were interesting?	0%	0%	0%	0%	100%	5.00
Do you feel that you learned anything new in the sessions?	0%	0%	5%	10%	85%	4.80
Did you feel that you could speak openly about your feelings towards the different topics discussed during the sessions?	0%	0%	15%	5%	80%	4.65
Do you think that participating in these sessions will help you in your job?	0%	0%	26%	21%	53%	4.26
Would you recommend this ethics education program to other nursing assistants?	0%	0%	0%	11%	89%	4.90
Would you want to go to more ethics sessions like this one in the future?	0%	5%	20%	15%	60%	4.30
Was it helpful to have the opportunity to discuss these issues with other nursing assistants?	0%	0%	5%	5%	90%	4.85
Did you like hearing what other nursing assistants had to say about these issues?	0%	0%	5%	45%	50%	4.45

power (or the doctor's power) to cure or keep the resident alive. Similarly, the majority of CNAs were confident that they were doing a good job. Fifty-eight percent reported "never" feeling that they are not doing their job well enough. During discussion, subjects said that when a resident is dying all you can do is care for the resident and provide comfort. CNAs generally felt confident that they do their best for residents.

While caring for dying residents can often be distressing, CNAs reported positive aspects to the work. The majority of CNAs "agreed" (59%) or "strongly agreed" (19%) that caring for dying residents can be a very rewarding experience. When CNAs were asked to elaborate on their responses to this question they said that while they receive few external rewards (e.g., money, praise, acknowledgments), they feel the work is spiritually rewarding and meaningful.

Fifty percent of subjects also "agreed" or "strongly agreed" that caring for dying residents can be a very rewarding experience, even if residents are dying because they refused to have a feeding tube. Here, however, there was significantly less agreement than when refusal of a feeding tube was not mentioned in the question (t = 2.47; p < .05). Similarly, about half the CNAs "agreed" (26%) or "strongly agreed" (22%) that is more difficult to care for residents who are dying because they are refusing a feeding tube than if they were dying from a disease over which they have no control.

Despite the fact that CNAs often found it more emotionally difficult to care for residents who were dying because they refused treatment, CNAs felt that these residents were entitled to good nursing home care. Almost all subjects (96%) "disagreed" or "strongly disagreed" that residents who do not want life-sustaining treatment should not be admitted to a nursing home. A similar percentage of subjects (92%) "disagreed" or "strongly disagreed" that they would rather not be assigned to residents who were dying because they refused a feeding tube.

SUPPORT GROUP SESSION DISCUSSIONS

The vast majority of time during the support sessions was devoted to the CNAs' discussion of their feelings, thoughts, and needs when caring for dying residents. One of the issues discussed was the current level of support provided to CNAs. CNAs felt that most support is provided by other nursing staff on the unit, including both CNAs and nurses. CNAs often said that the nurses also become attached to residents and are generally supportive and understanding when a resident dies. Support on the units is typically provided in an informal manner. Staff are generally considerate and protective of a CNA who loses a resident to whom he or she is close. While support was available to the CNAs on their respective nursing units, they felt they did not receive adequate support from the institution as a whole. Staff on individual units are left to cope on their own, a situation which can sometimes be difficult and inadequate. For example, one CNA said that recently there were a number of deaths on her floor and it was a distressing period for all of the nursing staff on the unit. No one came to see how the staff were coping, whether they needed extra support, or even asked how they were feeling. The CNA felt there was no acknowledgment or appreciation of the pain the staff was experiencing.

Some CNAs felt administration as well as other staff members think that caring for dying residents is "just a part of the job" and therefore no real consideration is given to providing them with support. An incident that illustrated this point occurred during one of the support sessions. One of the CNAs had missed the first support group session so the group facilitator provided the CNA with a brief overview of the program. Following the overview, the CNA said: "So this is to help the families?" The facilitator replied, "No, this is for you—to help you, the CNAs, because you work so closely with the residents." A second CNA then said: "Isn't it funny, there are always inservices about what's best for the residents or the families, but there is never anything for us." CNAs were frustrated that while they are repeatedly instructed on how to provide the best possible care to residents and families their own needs are rarely addressed.

In circumstances where support from outside staff has been available it was greatly appreciated. It is the policy at one of the facilities for the ethics committee to meet with staff caring for residents who are dying when life-sustaining treatment has been removed. CNAs said they appreciate this type of support. Additionally, one of the CNAs said that when she was particularly distressed by one of her cases, the director of nursing met with her and was very supportive. The CNA found this meeting to be very helpful. Thus, it appears that when support is offered it is valued and effective.

CNAs spent a good deal of time during the support sessions discussing the relationships they develop with residents. As was found in the larger educational study, CNAs said there is an understanding that staff are not supposed to get overly attached to residents. In support of this view, a few CNAs stated they maintain an emotional distance with residents specifically to protect themselves from the pain of losing someone about whom they care. One CNA said she used to get close to residents in the past, but tries not to anymore because it is so painful.

Most CNAs felt it is inevitable that they become attached to residents due to the extensive time they spend together. Moreover, many CNAs seemed to gain a great deal from their relationship with residents. They often considered residents to be like members of their families and similarly, they felt cared for and appreciated by residents.

CNAs discussed how they often went out of their way to provide comfort to distressed residents. One CNA described a resident who was angry and depressed about being admitted to a nursing home. The resident would not get out of bed and refused to eat the food provided. The CNA asked the resident what he would like to eat. The resident replied, "Sesame noodles and hot and sour soup." The CNA went to a restaurant outside of the nursing home and bought the food. The resident ate all of it. The CNA said that when his father was dying he tried to bring him things that he liked to eat. He provided that same consideration to the resident. A number of CNAs reported similar stories about bringing in outside food for residents in order to improve their quality of life.

Often caring is conveyed by small yet extremely thoughtful gestures. A CNA spoke about a resident she took care of who had lost the ability to communicate due to a stroke. The CNA was very fond of the resident and she knew the resident loved flowers so she used to always put a flower in the resident's button hole to make the resident feel good. Another CNA spoke about the special relationship she had with one of the residents on her unit who was not under her direct care. When the resident was dying the CNA went to her room, talked to her, and held her hand. She said she wanted to be there for the resident in the end and she felt good about it.

CNAs even become attached to their more difficult residents. One CNA said he takes care of a resident who swears all the time. The CNA said he didn't mind this because it was "kind of a man-to-man thing."

The caring relationship between CNAs and residents was often reciprocated. CNAs talked with pride about the strong attachment their residents have for them. They said they were often introduced by residents as if they were family members. A number of CNAs reported that their residents will refuse to let a different CNA bathe them. The resident will say, "Oh she doesn't give a bath the same way you do." Some residents will even refuse to have a bath when their regular CNA goes on vacation.

Some residents were also described as being considerate of CNAs' moods and feelings. CNAs said residents often sense when something is the matter. One CNA said one of her residents has said, "Oh you don't look so good. Save your strength. You can give me the bath tomorrow." The resident then reports to the nurse that she already had her bath in order to protect the CNA. Another CNA said one of her residents saves her a cookie and a can of ginger ale every evening so that she can have a little break. The CNAs are touched by these displays of caring, and are proud of the positive relationships that they have with residents.

In addition to the positive components of their job, CNAs talked about those things they find most difficult. Many CNAS discussed the deaths of residents for whom they cared.

While a close relationship with residents provided many positive things, the death of a favorite resident was described as painful. CNAs provided a number of examples illustrating these distressing experiences. One CNA said she found out her favorite resident died while she was on vacation. When she returned the head nurse told her, "Your baby died." The CNA said she was so upset she cried for two days. Similarly, another CNA said he was at home when one of his residents died and a coworker called to let him know. The CNA said that when he got off the phone he said to his wife, "One of my friends died."

When asked if they are ever sad when caring for their residents, another CNA said that he had cried earlier in the day when one of his residents had died unexpectedly. This was a resident he felt close to and would often go to for advice. The CNA described this resident as having been his mentor and the loss was considerable.

In addition to losing a resident to whom the CNA feels close, CNAs listed a number factors that can make a case particularly difficult. One such factor is dying and death of a resident with no family or friends to help provide comfort at the end of life. CNAs were very aware of the need to provide comfort to dying residents and they talked about their inability to spend a satisfactory amount of time with dying residents. Many said they wished they could spend more time with dying residents but that it isn't possible due to the limited number of staff and their responsibilities to other residents. One CNA said: "Dying residents always want someone to hold their hand and you just can't sit with them for too long because you have to take care of seven or eight other residents. Sometimes you wait until they fall asleep and then you sneak out of the room." CNAs said it is a comfort to them (as well as residents) when they know there is a friend or family member sitting with the resident.

CNAs sometimes expressed anger at families for not coming to visit their relatives or not spending enough time with them. When asked why they thought families sometimes do not come to visit, CNAs listed a variety of reasons. Some felt that families don't care enough about the residents, others felt families feel guilt over placing residents in a nursing home, or families don't want to see how the resident has deteriorated. Generally, CNAs felt that families should be as involved as possible and some suggested that nursing homes provide counseling for families to help them cope with the issues related to having a family member in a nursing home.

As discussed throughout this book, CNAs said they find it difficult when families decide a resident should not receive life-sustaining treatment, particularly a feeding tube. CNAs typically stated that if a resident does not want treatment the resident's wishes should be respected. They felt the resident was entitled to make these decisions about his or her own life. CNAs were upset, however, when they perceived that the family made the decision to end treatment. As one CNA put it: "If it's what the person wants that's good and I'm happy to take care of him, but 80 percent of the time it's the family who makes these decisions and I don't feel good about that." CNAs felt that it is as if the family is giving up on the resident when treatment is discontinued.

Many CNAs said they would prefer to see a resident get treatment. They said there have been cases of residents who were fed by feeding tube and then improved enough to eat by mouth. They believe it is important to give the residents the chance to recover. What makes this situation more difficult is that CNAs are often not included in the treatment decision-making process. For example, one CNA spoke about the following case. A resident could no longer eat and needed a feeding tube to stay alive. A decision was made not to insert a feeding tube. The CNA said she did not know what the resident's wishes were or whether he had a living-will stating that he did not want a feeding tube. What upset the CNA was that notes in the chart indicated that the daughter did not want a feeding tube inserted. The CNA said she would have felt much better if she knew this was what the resident wanted. In a similar situation, another CNA said he found out that a resident had an advance directive stating he did not want a feeding tube. The CNA said this made him feel much better about the decision not to insert the feeding tube.

One of the responsibilities that many CNAs reported as distressing was taking care of the resident's body after death. This was particularly difficult earlier in the CNAs' work experience. One CNA said the first time she had to clean the body of one of her residents she hid in the bathroom. She said the nurse was very understanding and had her watch someone else clean and wrap the body. A second CNA said the first time she washed a body she was working in a hospital and the body was of a 20 year-old boy. She said she kept seeing her son's face in place of the boy's. She stated that the boy's name would always be with her. Most CNAs, however, felt that cleaning and wrapping the body becomes somewhat easier with more experience. One CNA said wrapping the bodies affected her when she first started working, but now when a resident dies she just wraps the body and it is done. Other CNAs agreed that it gets easier, but can still be difficult when it is a resident they are close to.

Following the resident's death, CNAs also said they find it difficult to adjust to the fact that the bed is immediately filled with someone new. CNAs felt there is not adequate opportunity to mourn the death of the resident. Additionally, many believe the bed is immediately filled for financial gains and that this has become more important than respect for the resident after death. Some CNAs said it is difficult to think about starting a new relationship so soon after losing someone. There is a fear of going through the painful process yet again. One CNA said that she is very close to one of her residents and she knows that if this resident dies she will not feel as close to someone new placed in the room.

Although CNAs talked highly of their relationships with many family members who they felt were very appreciative of the work that they do, another difficulty associated with the job included CNAs' feelings that they are sometimes not treated well by families. Additionally, they said they generally only receive recognition from administration for the mistakes that they make, rather than for the good job that they do.

When asked about what are some of the things that CNAs do to help them cope with the difficulties of their job, many CNAs discussed the importance of religion in their lives. Religion was an important source of comfort and inspiration when working with the dying. Some CNAs also said they could discuss some things with their family members and that this was helpful as well. Overall, however, there were few things that CNAs said that they already did to alleviate their work-related stress and concerns.

CNAs were also asked whether there were things they felt that would help them with the distressing components of their work. Many said it would be helpful to go to the resident's funeral or memorial service. They felt they should be allowed to go and transportation should be provided. The CNAs said they want to be able to express their respect and caring for the resident and they feel this would be helpful to the families as well. Some CNAs said they would like the opportunity to help families after the death of a resident (e.g., cooking a meal for them). Similar to going to a funeral, this would give a degree of closure as well as provide the opportunity to show respect for the resident's memory.

Like the CNAs in the educational sessions, the CNAs in the support groups felt that it would be helpful to be included more regularly in discussions about resident care. They should be told about the resident's own treatment choices as early in the care-taking process as possible, if possible even before there is a medical crisis.

Many said that it would be a great help if families participated more in the care of residents. Families need to be there when the resident dies and there should be increased dialogues with the families to facilitate this. CNAs said when families are not there the CNAs feel they are not doing enough for the residents. They want to sit with the residents when the residents need them but they have too many other responsibilities to be able to do this. They would feel better if they knew the family was sitting in the room with the resident.

CNAs also felt that more education about what to expect on the job would be helpful. They said they are taught the mechanical components of the job, but they are not told about what to expect in terms of their emotional involvement and responses. Ongoing education about care of the dying was also something that CNAs would like the opportunity to have.

CNAs' Evaluations of the Program

As can be seen from TABLE 11.2, CNAs had very positive feelings about participating in the program. During the sessions the CNAs participated enthusiastically and shared their experiences with others. As in the educational sessions, they also appreciated the opportunity to hear their coworkers' opinions. One CNA said she was glad to have been part of these sessions because she was currently dealing with these same issues in her personal life. Her mother was in a nursing home and she had to make a decision about a feeding tube placement. This CNA felt it was extremely helpful to hear the opinions and experiences expressed by other CNAs and this helped her come to a decision. She said she now felt more comfortable allowing her mother to have a feeding tube. Another CNA said that she takes more time to think about the various factors that may have gone into a decision to continue or discontinue curative treatment. A further indication of the participating CNAs' enthusiasm for the program was that one of the CNAs brought in a journal article related to the topics discussed during the sessions.

The following are some of the CNAs' comments from the open-ended questions on the evaluation form:

"You learn how to deal with dying residents and their families."

"Other nursing assistants should have training on death and dying and other departments should know about the dying process."

"It's good to discuss your feelings openly. . . . This was a very good experience."

"I liked the discussions and opinions of other CNAs. . . . I think every CNA should attend one of these sessions."

"The time was too short."

"You learn how to relax."

"The sessions were very interesting and a learning experience."

"I found these sessions helped me make a personal decision about an important member of my family."

"I would like more inservices on the care and well-being of residents and staff."

"The meeting was very good for me. I learned more about comfort care and I got a chance to discuss problems about the residents. . . . Educational programs like these are very good for all of the nursing assistants."

"We could be frank and open about all matters."

"We should have more sessions, get family members involved more; too many residents, not enough staff, over-worked."

"What I liked most were the topics we discussed and especially discussing our feelings towards residents and their families."

"We have to give and do anything, as much as we can, to help the dying person because these are her/his final days."

"I liked most being able to speak openly."

"We should have more of these sessions."

DISCUSSION

The findings from these support groups indicate that CNAs often experience distress when caring for the dying. It is not surprising that CNAs reported feelings of sadness, stress, or hopelessness. These are normal responses in grief situations when one loses a meaningful person in one's life (e.g., Doka, 1989), and clearly someone the CNA has seen and cared for on a daily basis becomes meaningful. These findings, however, illustrate the need to address the thoughts and feelings of CNAs and provide them with the needed support.

While CNAs reported receiving support from nursing staff on their units, they did not feel adequately supported by the institution as a whole. Support from the individual units may be sufficient much of the time, but it can be draining on the limited emotional and physical resources of a unit, particularly when many of the staff within the unit are progressing through difficult situations at the same time.

Additionally, when support is only provided in an informal manner, it is easy for people to fall through the cracks without having their needs met. The most vocal CNAs or those with the most high profile or difficult cases will have the opportunity for support, while others may not. Support should be available in an on-going capacity so that burnout or crisis situations are avoided.

Our findings supported the hypothesis that CNAs find it more distressing to work with residents who were refusing a feeding tube (or other life-sustaining treatments) than with residents for which this was not an issue. There appeared to be a variety of reasons for this. Due to previous experience, CNAs were aware that residents who receive a feeding tube can occasionally improve and regain the ability to eat. They feel that the decision to stop or not start treatment is in effect giving up on the resident. Additionally, CNAs feel that the majority of time that these types of decisions are made, it is family rather than resident preferences that are being favored. Inclusion of CNAs in treatment care planning can address both of these issues. It can be made clear to CNAs that it is the resident's wishes that are being supported. Additionally, it can be explained that while there may be some conditions that can be reversed with the use of a feeding tube, other conditions exist that make the chance of recovery extremely slim, and it is the resident's choice not to extend their life with excessive treatment such as a feeding tube.

Despite the fact that CNAs sometimes said they were upset by a decision not to continue aggressive medical treatment, the great majority did not object to working with residents who refused life-sustaining treatment. Similarly, the majority felt residents should be admitted to a nursing home even if they are refusing life-sustaining treatment. CNAs felt that even residents who refuse curative treatment can still benefit from comfort care. This is an important and accurate point and one that should be encouraged and positively reinforced.

CNAs were positive about their experience in this type of support program. They were enthusiastic about discussing their own experiences of working with dying residents and they valued the opportunity to listen to other CNAs' thoughts and feelings. It was especially important to CNAs to feel that their opinions were important and their work is crucial to the nursing home. It is important to keep this in mind and to praise CNAs for the good work that they do on an ongoing basis, not only during distressing situations.

It should be pointed out that the subjects who took part in this study were chosen by nursing management specifically for this project. Thus, there may have been a selection bias in the sample with nurses choosing those CNAs who they felt would enjoy and benefit from this type of program. Further studies need to examine the impact of support programs for all participating CNAs in a facility. It is possible that not all CNAs will benefit from the same type of supportive program. Additionally, support programs such as this may only be one part of a comprehensive system that needs to be in place to support both CNAs and other on-line staff. Different options need to be explored and available for the various needs of staff.

This project only involved participation for five weekly one-hour sessions. Longer term support programs need to be examined along with additional outcome measures such as job satisfaction, employment turnover, work-related stress, and especially resident care.

REFERENCES

Doka, K. J. (1989). *Disenfranchised grief.* Lexington, MA: Lexington Books.
Lerea, L. E., & LiMauro, B. F. (1982). Grief among healthcare workers: A comparative study. *Journal of Gerontology, 37*(5), 604–608.
Lev, E. (1989). A nurse's perspective on disenfranchised grief. In K. Doka (Ed.), *Disenfranchised grief* (pp. 287–299). Lexington, MA: D. C. Health.
Sheard, T. (1984). Dealing with the nurse's grief. *Nursing Forum*(1), 43–45.
Robbins, I., Lloyd, C., Carpenster, S., & Bender, M. P. (1992). Staff anxieties about death in residential facilities for elderly people. *Journal of Advanced Nursing, 17,* 548–553.
Sonstegard, L., Hansen, N., Zillman, L., & Johnson, M. K. (1976). The grieving nurse. *American Journal of Nursing, 76*(9), 1490–1492.
Wilson, S. A., & Daley, B. J. (1998). Attachment/detachment: Forces influencing care of the dying in long-term care. *Journal of Palliative Medicine, 1*(1), 21–34.

12

Implications of the Project: Where Do We Go from Here?

We began this study with the belief that CNAs are the foundation of the long term care system and, in many instances, the most important people in the everyday lives of nursing home residents. We also believe that if we are to enable CNAs to function at the highest level possible and to maximize their ability to provide quality care, they must be treated as the valuable people that they are. This means they need the educational and emotional support necessary to carry out their important jobs. They must be treated as integral to resident care, and they must be given the respect they deserve for the work they do.

Many of us in the nursing home industry may believe that we do appreciate the importance of CNAs, and that we do treat them with the utmost respect and consideration. This project led us to believe, however, that CNAs generally do not feel this is the case. In fact, one of the surprising features of this project was the disparity between what administrative level personnel in nursing homes think of CNAs, and what CNAs believe the administrators think.

A criterion for a respective nursing home's participation in this project was the administrator's approval of the project. To obtain this, we sent an introductory letter to the nursing homes, asking to speak with the administrator. This was followed by a meeting between project staff and the administrator of the facility in the smaller homes, and between the project staff and nursing administration in the larger homes. Universally, one of the primary reasons for a facility's opting to participate in the project was the perception by these administrators that CNAs are extremely vital to the functioning of the home. They also expressed the concern that, while CNAs attend a number of mandatory inservices, they are so often left out of the loop on issues such as the ones we addressed as part of this project.

An obvious implication of all of this is the industry-wide need for facilities to develop mechanisms to make CNAs feel recognized, respected, and a part of the team at all levels of assessment and care. Any mechanisms that can be developed to accomplish this will be an improvement over the current state of affairs.

The other main areas that need to be addressed fall into the categories of education and emotional support. As noted in the description of the educational intervention used in this project, the areas of instruction we found most helpful centered on the ethical principles generally applied in health care settings, and the appropriate use of comfort care at the end of life. As well, we emphasized to the CNAs that they are vital members of the health care team.

RESPECTING RESIDENT AUTONOMY: WHAT DOES THIS MEAN FOR THE CNA?

The ethical principle of respect for autonomy, as noted earlier, is considered the basis of current biomedical ethics. The supposition in the United States is that we all have the right to be thoroughly informed about our medical conditions, and we have the right to make any and all decisions about treatment. This is respect for autonomy in action. However, allowing individuals to make autonomous choices in the long term care setting is often a challenge. In contrast to a younger population whose members are more likely to be able to articulate their treatment wishes, the principle of respect for autonomy is sometimes difficult to apply when dealing with a frail, elderly clientele. Although advance directives are the mechanism through which individuals can exercise autonomy in the event of diminished decision-making capacity, the use of advance directives is a relatively new and not yet particularly widespread phenomenon, although increasing numbers of adults are executing them.

In many situations in nursing homes, well-meaning families speak for the nursing home resident, and the CNAs seem to believe that it is perfectly appropriate for families to be doing this. In their own personal situations, CNAs say they would like their families to make decisions for them. However, on occasion, families may be making requests about treatment that staff (and particularly paraprofessional staff) may interpret as being the wishes of the family, and not the preferences of the resident. While most families clearly have the best interests of the resident at heart, CNAs often have difficulty when families request the limitation of life-sustaining treatment. Efforts must be made to explain to the CNAs that the family in this instance *is* speaking for the resident, and this is a form of extended autonomy.

When nursing home residents are still able to make their own decisions, stress needs to be placed on the fact that the wishes of the resident take precedence over the wishes of the family. Thus, while it may be difficult for caregivers to accept, residents who are cognitively intact have the right to make their own decisions, as well as the right to know their diagnoses and prognoses. Families, while integral to the lives of the resident, really do not have the right to overrule residents' choices, nor to make decisions about residents' care without the knowledge of the resident. While this concept may be difficult for all CNAs to accept, it may be even more difficult for those from cultures where individual autonomy is far less dominant. These CNAs may need extra attention and education about these issues on a regular basis.

COMFORT CARE: THE ROLE OF THE CNA

One of the most important components of this project was to educate CNAs about end-of-life care and their roles in providing it. This was a unique challenge, particularly when the end-of-life is associated with the exercise of patient autonomy involving the limitation of life-sustaining treatment. CNAs, like their professional counterparts, work in a health care environment where cure has long been the goal. This emphasis has become even more dominant as medical technology has enabled us to keep people alive far longer than ever before. Even in the long term care setting, where the majority of residents are clearly in their final years, health care providers may have difficulty accepting that the end is near. Accordingly, they see the use of life-sustaining treatment as appropriate in nearly every instance, and it is the rare occasion when one hears staff saying it is acceptable to just "let someone go."

Decisions to limit the use of life-sustaining treatment usually have a profound effect on the caregiving staff in nursing homes. In concert with the pervasive "cure" philosophy, there is the emotional effect of anticipating the loss of a resident with whom the CNA has established a long, close relationship. Additionally, there is the perception that once we opt not to use life-sustaining treatments, there is "nothing" to be done for the resident.

Unfortunately, the use of comfort care at the end of life is generally not perceived as being the caregiving equivalent of feeding tubes and IVs. This is a perception that is changing all too slowly. The national trend toward applying palliative care principles in an increasing number of situations is clearly growing. However, it has been relatively slow to gain a foothold in the long term care setting, despite the growing number of nursing homes with hospice contracts. In addition to some reimbursement issues precluding hospice use, this may be because while almost all patients who have a six-month prognosis as a result of most any disease are appropriate for hospice, the majority of hospice patients have cancer diagnoses. Cancer patients have historically been viewed as the "typical" hospice patient, but these individuals are in the minority in nursing homes. Rather, we see a large number of residents with dementia. While guidelines do exist for establishing a prognosis in dementing illnesses, generally dementia is a condition that physicians find difficult to prognosticate. Thus, although some (Volicer, Rheaume, Brown, Fabiszewski, & Brady, 1986) suggested using hospice principles for dementia patients more than ten years ago, the majority of patients with these conditions are referred to hospice programs relatively infrequently.

The view of comfort care as less important than medical technology is clearly a perception we would like to change, and the change needs to be system-wide. For now, we can begin to take steps to try to change the mind-set of our paraprofessional workforce, and encourage belief in the philosophy that comfort care in end-stage disease is as important if not more important than the use of medical technologies. Emphasis should be placed on those areas of comfort care in which CNAs play the most prominent role: mouth care, turning and positioning, hand-holding and talking to the resident. CNAs should also be instructed that adequate pain management is an achievable goal in nursing homes.

Another area associated with comfort care where CNAs (as well as their professional counterparts) need educational support centers on the dynamics associated with withholding or withdrawing life-sustaining treatment. The literature available on the impact of withholding or withdrawing artificial nutrition and hydration, while helpful and probably generalizable to a nursing home population, is mostly drawn from hospice work (Andrews & Levine, 1989; Billings, 1985; Printz, 1992; Zerwekh, 1987, 1997). The study conducted by Robert McCann and his colleagues (1994), however, describing their work with nursing home residents who were able to communicate and had opted to not receive feeding tubes and IVs, gives empirical evidence that dying without artificial nutrition and hydration is a comfortable experience.

The development of reading materials appropriate for the long term care industry's paraprofessional workforce would be most useful. What became obvious from our work with the CNAs in this project is that many of their opinions on care at the end of life are based on assumptions (e.g., what it must be like to "starve to death"). Conducting inservices and repeatedly reinforcing to the CNAs that terminal dehydration is strongly believed to be a comfortable process may not be enough. Much of what has been written in the medical and nursing journals is at a reading level that is very likely not to be comprehensible to the average CNA (while there is great variation in background among CNAs, many have limited reading skills or do not use English as their primary language). The development of user-friendly reading material on comfort care for CNAs could be a useful educational supplement (see "The CNA's Ethics Booklet" in the Appendix of the accompanying work-book as an example). As well, it might help assuage the emotional concerns of CNAs that dying without nutrition and hydration is a painful experience.

EDUCATION IN DEATH AND DYING

A related area where education for CNAs is desirable centers on death and dying. As noted in the evaluations of the education sessions, this is an area in which CNAs repeatedly requested more inservices. Dealing with the myriad issues surrounding this phenomenon can only be helpful to CNAs, many of whom had never seen a dead person before they began this work, let alone had the experience of caring for someone who is dying.

Interestingly, even though many CNAs come from cultures where death is less "sterilized" than it is in mainstream U.S. culture, the prospect of death is still frightening to them. There also needs to be some focus on dealing with loss. The phenomenon of caregiver grief is unique, and does not fit other bereavement models (see, for example, Doka, 1989). This is a key factor to recognize when dealing with the many losses that CNAs experience. Not only do they experience the loss of residents to whom they may have become particularly close, they also lose whatever relationship they had had with the resident's family. They often identify with the family's pain.

Another related issue that can potentially impact upon CNAs, particularly those from other countries and whose families do not live here, is the uncomfortable feeling associated with caring for other people's parents when geographical distance prevents one from caring for one's own.

THE CNA AS PART OF THE HEALTH CARE TEAM

An issue that repeatedly arose during the sessions as being distressing to the CNAs was their perceived exclusion as members of the health care team. They clearly recognized their importance, but felt than no one else did. In fact, they generally agreed that other members of the health care team (nurses, social workers, physicians, etc.) should be informed how important the role of the CNA was; their sense was they themselves already knew it. Any mechanism that nursing homes can develop to change the perceptions of other health care providers to realize the key role played by CNAs can only serve to enhance teamwork and as a result, improve resident care.

One concrete step that will integrate CNAs into the team to a greater degree is to involve them in all aspects of the treatment plan, including regular participation in team meetings where the patients to whom they are assigned are being discussed. When treatments that will be administered by CNAs are ordered, they will be carried out much more effectively if the CNA understands the reason for the treatment. For example, if a CNA is asked to apply a particular cream, it is helpful to her/him to understand what the cream is and what it is expected to accomplish. CNAs repeatedly told us they were told to do things, but rarely told why they were doing them.

It may also be helpful not only to the CNA but also to the overall care plan for a particular resident if particular treatments that will be administered by the CNA are analyzed in the context of the goals of treatment. For example, as noted earlier, as well as in the workbook accompanying this volume, one of the things that distressed CNAs was being made to get a resident out of bed when it was thought that the resident was more uncomfortable out of bed. CNAs regularly reported that if they were reluctant to get the resident up, it was thought by the nurse that the reason was the CNA's laziness. A discussion with the nurse about just why the CNA did not want to get the resident out of bed might result in reconsidering what was originally being done. Is it really necessary for this resident's well-being that she/he be gotten out of bed, or could they be kept equally (or perhaps even more) comfortable in bed?

SUPPORT FOR CNAS: A ROLE FOR CLERGY

And finally, given the relationship we found between many issues and the degree of religiosity felt by the CNA, it might be helpful for facilities to seek some support from clergy for their CNAs. Clergy of various denominations can fulfill this role, and often have a great deal of credibility with CNAs who are particularly religious. Using clergy to reassure CNAs about not only the importance of their work, but also the rightness and worth of their work, may be extremely beneficial to the CNAs.

CONCLUSION

Obviously, much more research on CNAs would be useful. Nonetheless, in conducting this project, as noted earlier, we did develop an extensive database of what CNAs know and think about ethical issues and end-of-life decision-making. Participation in the educational program did result in significant increases in knowledge about these issues, and may have raised the consciousness of CNAs about ethical issues at the end of life, both in the work arena and in their personal lives. The overwhelmingly positive responses to the program on the part of its participants was clearly a plus. The evaluations of the program also suggest that participation in programs of this nature may enhance the self-esteem of CNAs.

This program is clearly replicable in other nursing homes, and the training manual that accompanies this volume will enable other facilities to conduct the project on their own.

There were a number of issues we took as givens in planning this project. We were very aware going into it that CNAs provide the bulk of hands-on care, as well as the majority of emotional support, to frail elderly in nursing homes. We also knew they were excluded from many aspects of resident care, at least as far as inclusion in the care planning process and involvement in many of the psychosocial issues key to comprehensive care of the resident.

What we did not know was the extent to which this occurs, and the impact it has on the CNAs. Most disturbing, perhaps, is the lost potential that results from disempowering CNAs to the degree we do in the long term care industry. Clearly, given our conversations with many administrators and nursing directors, they *do* perceive the role of CNAs as extremely significant. Attempts must be made to make this perception of CNAs the universal perception, a view shared not only by a limited number of individuals but by all employed in the industry, as well as by families and future nursing home residents who will be cared for by these individuals.

We are also not so naive as to think that all CNAs are perfect. We are very aware that nursing home residents are subjected to verbal and, in some instances, physical abuse by nursing assistants (see, for example, Pillemer & Moore, 1989). And unfortunately, it is usually only this negative information that receives media attention. Nonetheless, we found a significant number of CNAs to be extremely kind, compassionate individuals performing emotionally and physically difficult tasks and regularly rising to this challenge. We hope that by disseminating the findings of this project, more nursing homes will implement this ethics program for CNAs. We also hope it will bring to the attention of the long term care industry and those who use its services the worth and the plight of the CNAs, and in so doing, enhance the quality of care delivered to frail elderly in nursing homes.

REFERENCES

Andrews, M. R., & Levine, A. M. (1989). Dehydration in the terminal patient: Perception of hospice nurses. *American Journal of Hospice Care, 6*, 31–34.

Billings, J. A. (1985). Comfort measures for the terminally ill: Is dehydration painful? *Journal of the American Geriatrics Society, 33*(11), 808–810.

Doka, K. J. (1989). *Disenfranchised grief.* Lexington, MA: D.C. Heath and Company.

McCann, R. M., Hall, W. J., & Groth-Juncker, A. (1994). Comfort care for terminally ill patients: The appropriate use of nutrition and hydration. *Journal of the American Medical Association, 272*(16), 1263–1266.

Pillemer, K., & Moore, D. W. (1989). Abuse of patients in nursing homes. *The Gerontologist, 29*(3), 314–320.

Printz, L. A. (1992). Terminal dehydration: A compassionate treatment. *Archives of Internal Medicine, 152*, 690–700.

Volicer, L., Rheaume, Y., Brown, J., Fabiszewski, K., & Brady, R. (1986). Hospice approach for the treatment of patients with advanced dementia of the Alzheimer's type. *Journal of the American Geriatrics Society, 42*(6), 597–603.

Zerwekh, J. V. (1987). Should fluid and nutritional support be withheld from terminally ill patients? *American Journal of Hospice Care, 4*(4), 37–38.

Zerwekh, J. V. (1997). Do dying patients really need IV fluids? *American Journal of Nursing, 97*(4), 37–38.

APPENDIXES

Appendix A

Responses in Percentages to All Knowledge and Attitude Questions on the Pretest and Posttest

PRETEST

Knowledge Questions (Percentage Responses)	YES	NO	DON'T KNOW	MISSING
6.[1] Can a health care proxy give someone the power to make financial decisions for the resident?	54.4	21.2	20.8	3.6
7. Can a health care proxy give someone the power to tell the doctor not to give the resident antibiotics when the resident has pneumonia?	54.8	23.9	17.0	4.4
8. Can a health care proxy give someone the power to sell the resident's home or apartment?	34.2	40.5	20.7	4.5
9. Can a health care proxy give someone the power to ask the doctor to stop a tube feeding once it has already begun?	56.1	23.9	16.2	3.9
10. Can a health care proxy give someone the power to ask the doctor not to start tube feeding if the resident is no longer taking food by mouth?	60.1	20.4	14.1	5.5
11. Can a health care proxy give someone the ability to sign permission for an amputation if the resident has gangrene?	59.3	19.1	16.8	4.8
12. If a resident left instructions (made out a living will) that he would not want to be fed by feeding tube if he could no longer swallow food and would never regain the ability to swallow food, can the nursing home give him a feeding tube anyway?	8.6	82.6	5.8	3.1
13. If a resident left instructions (made out a living will) that she would not want to have any amputa-	10.2	78.8	6.6	4.4

---

[1]Question number on the Ethics Questionnaire

tions, can a doctor perform an amputation if the patient gets gangrene?

14. If there is no living will and no health care proxy can the family make the decision to stop a feeding tube?	66.9	22.8	7.1	3.2
15. If there is no living will and no health care proxy can the doctor make a decision to stop a feeding tube?	51.5	32.5	12.6	3.4

Attitude Questions	Always	Some-times	Never	Don't Know	Missing
16. At this nursing home, do you think that:					
a. the staff tries to find out what kinds of treatment very sick residents want?	50.6	28.9	5.7	11.1	3.8
b. when residents become ill, they or their health care proxy are told about the different choices they have as far as different types of treatments are concerned?	63.3	16.0	1.3	15.0	4.3
c. when residents become ill, they or their health care proxy are helped to make a decision about their treatment?	53.2	22.0	2.7	17.1	5.0
d. families of residents who are dying get some kind of emotional support or counseling?	54.8	23.9	3.4	0.0	18.0
e. staff, who are caring for residents who are dying, get some kind of emotional support or counseling?	17.6	26.0	41.8	9.7	4.9

17. **Sometimes situations exist in nursing homes that make it difficult to make decisions about the care given to residents who are very sick or terminally ill. How much do you think each of the following keeps the staff in this nursing home from being able to make decisions about care? (Circle the number that best describes what you think.)**

	NOT AT ALL	SOME-WHAT	VERY MUCH	MISSING
a. differences of opinion among staff	28.1	44.9	16.2	10.8
b. lack of knowledge about all the possible choices that could be made	28.9	38.8	15.1	17.3

c. not including all staff in the decisions about treatment	30.7	29.9	24.7	14.7
d. fear of being sued	22.1	27.1	32.3	18.5
e. how much something will cost	32.0	28.1	18.3	21.6
f. not enough staff	19.9	24.9	38.9	16.4
g. communication problems among the staff	22.6	36.8	26.8	13.7
h. communication problems with residents or their families	27.1	39.3	20.8	12.7

	DISAGREE	AGREE	DON'T KNOW	MISSING
18. Sometimes it is right *not to start* a treatment, such as a feeding tube, even if it means a resident might die sooner.	49.3	34.9	12.0	3.8
19. Sometimes it is right to *stop* a treatment, such as a feeding tube, even if it means a resident may die sooner.	54.9	29.9	11.8	3.4
20. A dying person should always be offered food and water by mouth.	37.6	52.2	7.6	2.6
21. A dying person should always receive food and water, even by feeding tube if necessary.	28.4	61.6	7.3	2.7
22. Sometimes we make dying residents more uncomfortable by continuing to give them food and water by mouth than if we didn't.	26.7	55.6	14.7	3.1
23. Sometimes we make dying residents more uncomfortable by giving them tube feedings and IVs than if we didn't feed them.	38.0	42.0	16.2	3.9
24. If you talk to a resident about a DNR (Do Not Resuscitate) order they will think their condition is hopeless.	38.6	42.3	14.1	5.0
25. All residents who are able to make decisions for themselves have the right to refuse life-saving treatment, even if refusing such treatment may result in death.	6.0	88.4	2.6	3.1
26. Many residents prefer to let other people make decisions for them.	32.8	52.0	11.6	3.6
27. Letting a patient die by not giving them a certain treatment is the same thing as helping them to commit suicide.	34.4	52.8	8.4	4.4
28. Some residents or their families have sued doctors when the residents were given a	14.2	58.5	22.9	4.4

treatment to keep them alive that they did not want.

29. It is possible to prevent dying residents from feeling much pain.	19.7	63.3	13.1	3.9
30. Discontinuing a feeding tube is the same as killing a resident.	53.3	33.1	11.5	2.1
31. Sometimes it is right to give pain medication to relieve suffering, even if it will make a person die sooner.	28.6	53.3	15.0	3.1
32. Many patients prefer not to know they are dying.	15.7	72.7	10.2	1.4
33. If a resident is suffering from some condition that causes him or her to be unable to make a decision (for example, Alzheimer's disease), the *doctor* is the best person to make decisions for the resident.	48.6	40.1	8.9	2.4
34. If a resident is suffering from some condition that causes him or her to be unable to make a decision (for example, Alzheimer's disease), a *family member* is the best person to make decisions for the resident.	16.2	73.0	8.2	2.6
35. We should not use expensive treatments to keep very old people alive.	81.3	7.9	9.0	1.7
36. In this nursing home the spiritual needs of dying residents receive too little attention.	54.4	29.9	12.4	3.2
37. My opinions about what should be done for residents are valued by the people I work with.	33.6	46.0	13.7	6.6
38. I am not comfortable caring for residents who will most likely die because *they* are refusing life-sustaining treatment.	72.1	16.6	7.4	3.9
39. I am not comfortable caring for residents who will most likely die because *their health care proxies* are refusing life-sustaining treatment.	63.2	21.3	10.7	4.8
40. Sometimes I feel the treatments we give the residents are too uncomfortable for them.	44.3	39.6	13.2	3.0
41. If a resident wants antibiotics in order to be kept alive the nursing home should provide them.	9.7	75.6	11.8	2.9
42. If a resident wants a feeding tube in order to be kept alive the nursing home should provide it.	8.4	82.1	6.0	3.6

43. If a resident does not want antibiotics and wants to die, the nursing home should not force treatment upon the resident.   10.5   79.3   7.1   3.0

44. If a resident does not want tube feeding and wants to die, the nursing home should not force the treatment upon the resident.   9.0   82.7   6.0   2.2

45. It is wrong to stop antibiotics, if it will keep the resident alive, even if the resident doesn't want it.   45.9   34.1   13.1   6.9

46. It is wrong to stop a feeding tube, if it will keep the resident alive, even if the resident doesn't want it.   44.3   37.0   11.5   7.3

47. If a family asks us not to tell a resident, *who can understand,* that he or she has an illness and a certain amount of time to live, we should go along with the family's request and not tell the resident.   17.3   70.3   9.7   2.8

48. **Sometimes, nursing assistants have the chance to discuss a resident's illness and treatment with other staff members, the resident, and/or the resident's family. Please circle the number that best describes how satisfied you are with the opportunities you have to discuss residents' treatment with each of the following people.**

		Not satisfied	Somewhat satisfied	Very satisfied	Missing
a.	physicians	38.8	21.8	18.7	20.6
b.	nurses	16.2	36.3	35.4	12.2
c.	social workers	30.2	28.4	21.8	19.5
d.	clergy	41.0	17.9	12.4	28.6
e.	administrators	39.7	21.8	13.4	25.0
f.	residents	28.8	27.0	24.1	20.2
g.	residents' families	28.8	31.5	19.7	20.0

49. At this nursing home, who do you think most often makes the final decision for mentally impaired residents who might need to be fed by feeding tubes and IVs?

FAMILY	DOCTOR	BOTH	OTHER	MISSING
38.6	33.6	20.0	2.6	5.2

50. Who do you think should make the final decision for mentally impaired residents who might need to be fed by feeding tubes and IVs?

FAMILY	DOCTOR	BOTH	OTHER	MISSING
42.3	32.3	18.3	2.2	4.9

51. Do you think the family should be able to make decisions about treatment when there is no health care proxy and no living will?

YES	NO	MISSING
82.2	12.9	4.9

52. Do you agree that when residents are capable of making decisions concerning life-threatening conditions (for example, if they have pneumonia but ask not to be treated with antibiotics), that their families should be able to overrule the resident's decision?

YES	NO	MISSING
29.6	64.6	5.8

POSTTEST

Knowledge Questions (Percentage Responses)	YES	NO	DON'T KNOW	MISSING
6.[2] Can a health care proxy give someone the power to make financial decisions for the resident?	53.7	31.8	13.8	0.7
7. Can a health care proxy give someone the power to tell the doctor not to give the resident antibiotics when the resident has pneumonia?	64.0	24.3	11.2	0.4
8. Can a health care proxy give someone the power to sell the resident's home or apartment?	34.1	48.6	16.4	0.9
9. Can a health care proxy give someone the power to ask the doctor to stop a tube feeding once it has already begun?	61.2	23.8	13.1	1.9
10. Can a health care proxy give someone the power to ask the doctor not to start tube feeding if the resident is no longer taking food by mouth?	67.8	19.4	9.3	3.5
11. Can a health care proxy give someone the ability to sign permission for an amputation if the resident has gangrene?	66.1	16.1	14.0	3.7
12. If a resident left instructions (made out a living will) that he would not want to be fed by feeding tube if he could no longer swallow food and would never re-	6.8	84.3	5.4	3.5

[2]Question number on the Ethics Questionnaire

gain the ability to swallow food, can the nursing home give him a feeding tube anyway?				
13. If a resident left instructions (made out a living will) that she would not want to have any amputations, can a doctor perform an amputation if the patient gets gangrene?	9.1	79.7	7.7	3.5
14. If there is no living will and no health care proxy, can the family make the decision to stop a feeding tube?	64.3	25.7	7.9	2.1
15. If there is no living will and no health care proxy, can the doctor make a decision to stop a feeding tube?	52.6	30.6	14.7	2.1

Attitude Questions	**Always**	**Some-times**	**Never**	**Don't Know**	**Missing**
16e. At this nursing home, do you think that staff, who are caring for residents who are dying, get some kind of emotional support or counseling?	17.3	30.4	35.3	14.3	2.8

	DISAGREE	**AGREE**	**DON'T KNOW**	**MISSING**
20. A dying person should always be offered food and water by mouth.	34.3	58.2	5.1	2.4
21. A dying person should always receive food and water, even by feeding tube if necessary.	30.8	60.0	6.8	2.3
24. If you talk to a resident about a DNR (Do Not Resuscitate) order, they will think their condition is hopeless.	38.8	42.3	17.1	1.8
25. All residents who are able to make decisions for themselves have the right to refuse life-saving treatment, even if refusing such treatment may result in death.	6.1	89.0	4.0	0.9
26. Many residents prefer to let other people make decisions for them.	39.3	47.0	12.4	1.4
27. Letting a patient die by not giving them a certain treatment is the same thing as helping them to commit suicide.	40.7	48.1	9.8	1.4
28. Some residents or their families have sued doctors when the residents were given a	14.0	54.4	28.5	3.1

treatment to keep them alive that they
did not want.

29. It is possible to prevent dying residents from feeling much pain.	15.7	69.6	11.3	2.8
30. Discontinuing a feeding tube is the same as killing a resident.	57.0	29.7	11.2	2.1
31. Sometimes it is right to give pain medication to relieve suffering, even if it will make a person die sooner.	22.7	60.0	14.7	2.5
32. Many patients prefer not to know they are dying.	16.6	74.3	7.5	1.6
33. If a resident is suffering from some condition that causes him or her to be unable to make a decision (for example, Alzheimer's disease), the *doctor* is the best person to make decisions for the resident.	49.8	40.9	8.2	1.2
34. If a resident is suffering from some condition that causes him or her to be unable to make a decision (for example, Alzheimer's disease), a *family member* is the best person to make decisions for the resident.	16.8	74.5	5.6	3.1
36. In this nursing home the spiritual needs of dying residents receive too little attention.	53.7	29.4	15.7	1.2
37. My opinions about what should be done for residents are valued by the people I work with.	30.1	48.1	17.8	4.0
38. I am not comfortable caring for residents who will most likely die because *they* are refusing life-sustaining treatment.	60.3	10.3	5.4	24.0
39. I am not comfortable caring for residents who will most likely die because *their health care proxies* are refusing life-sustaining treatment.	55.4	13.1	7.0	24.5
40. Sometimes I feel the treatments we give the residents are too uncomfortable for them.	48.6	34.8	13.8	2.8
41. If a resident wants antibiotics in order to be kept alive the nursing home should provide them.	10.7	75.7	12.1	1.4
42. If a resident wants a feeding tube in order to be kept alive the nursing home should provide it.	8.2	80.4	9.1	2.4
43. If a resident does not want antibiotics and wants to die, the nursing home should not force the treatment upon the resident.	11.0	79.2	7.9	1.9

44. If a resident does not want tube feeding   19.7   79.4   7.9   1.8
    and wants to die, the nursing home
    should not force the treatment upon
    the resident.

47. If a family asks us not to tell a resident,   19.4   71.5   7.2   1.8
    who can understand, that he or she has an
    illness and a certain amount of time to
    live, we should go along with the family's
    request and not tell the resident.

48. **Sometimes, nursing assistants have the chance to discuss a resident's illness and treat-
    ment with other staff members, the resident, and/or the resident's family. Please circle
    the number that best describes how satisfied you are with the opportunities you have
    to discuss residents' treatment with each of the following people.**

		Not satisfied	Somewhat satisfied	Very satisfied	Missing
a.	physicians	38.8	23.8	19.2	18.3
b.	nurses	14.7	35.3	38.6	11.4
c.	social workers	34.6	27.3	20.1	18.0
d.	clergy	46.3	18.9	11.4	23.3
c.	administrators	47.0	20.3	8.4	24.3
f.	residents	28.3	28.5	18.5	24.8
g.	residents' families	28.5	30.1	20.8	20.6

49. At this nursing home, who do you think most often makes the final decision for
    mentally impaired residents who might need to be fed by feeding tubes and IVs?

FAMILY	DOCTOR	BOTH	OTHER	MISSING
43.7	43.0	9.3	2.6	1.4

50. Who do you think should make the final decision for mentally impaired residents who
    might need to be fed by feeding tubes and IVs?

FAMILY	DOCTOR	BOTH	OTHER	MISSING
46.5	40.4	9.1	1.9	2.1

51. Do you think the family should be able to make decisions about treatment when there
    is no health care proxy and no living will?

YES	NO	MISSING
84.3	14.3	1.4

52. Do you agree that when residents are capable of making decisions concerning life-
    threatening conditions (for example, if they have pneumonia but ask not to be treated
    with antibiotics), that their families should be able to overrule the resident's decision?

YES	NO	MISSING
29.0	67.3	3.7

Appendix B
The Ethics Education Evaluation Form

ETHICS EDUCATION EVALUATION FORM

Please circle the number which best describes how you feel about each of the following questions.

1. Do you feel that you personally needed these sessions?

NOT AT ALL		SOME-WHAT		VERY MUCH
1	2	3	4	5

2. Do you feel that other nursing assistants in the group needed the sessions?

NOT AT ALL		SOME-WHAT		VERY MUCH
1	2	3	4	5

3. Do you think the sessions were interesting?

NOT AT ALL		SOME-WHAT		VERY MUCH
1	2	3	4	5

4. Do you feel that you learned anything new in the sessions?

NOT AT ALL		SOME-WHAT		VERY MUCH
1	2	3	4	5

5. Did you feel that you could speak openly about your feelings towards the different topics discussed during the sessions?

NOT AT ALL		SOME-WHAT		VERY MUCH
1	2	3	4	5

6. Do you think that participating in these sessions will help you in your job?

NOT AT ALL		SOME-WHAT		VERY MUCH
1	2	3	4	5

7. Would you recommend this ethics education program to other nursing assistants?

NOT AT ALL		SOME- WHAT		VERY MUCH
1	2	3	4	5

8. Would you want to go to more ethics sessions like this one in the future?

NOT AT ALL		SOME- WHAT		VERY MUCH
1	2	3	4	5

9. Was it helpful to have the opportunity to discuss these issues with other nursing assistants?

NOT AT ALL		SOME- WHAT		VERY MUCH
1	2	3	4	5

10. Did you like hearing what other nursing assistants had to say about these issues?

NOT AT ALL		SOME- WHAT		VERY MUCH
1	2	3	4	5

What did you like most about the sessions? _____
_____
_____

What did you like least about the sessions? _____
_____
_____

Are there any topics that you think we should have discussed that were not discussed at all or were not discussed in enough detail? _____
_____
_____

Please write down any comments, suggestions, or complaints: _____
_____
_____

As a nursing assistant, what types of inservices or educational programs do you think would be most valuable to you? _____
_____
_____

Thank you very much for your participation in this program! It has been a pleasure working with all of you!

Index

Page numbers followed by "t" indicate tables.

Teaching End-of-Life Ethics to CNAs

Orah R. Burack, MA
Eileen R. Chichin, PhD, RN
Ellen Olson, MD

 Springer Publishing Company

Contents

Appendixes

PART I

A GUIDE TO THE PROGRAM

1

Introduction

This educational program was originally conducted with over 600 CNAs from 28 nursing homes throughout New York and New Jersey, with the generous support of the Greenwall Foundation. The project emerged from two areas of interest. The first is the current emphasis within medical ethics on patient and resident autonomy concerning treatment decision-making. The second is the central yet often overlooked role of the certified nursing assistant within the health care team. The goal of this project is to educate certified nursing assistants (CNAs) in end-of-life ethical issues such as patient autonomy, advance directives, family and patient decision-making, and comfort care. Additionally, a key objective is to provide a supportive environment for CNAs to discuss their thoughts and feelings about care of the dying. The intention of this workbook is to enable nursing homes to conduct an ethics education program within their own facilities.

2

Background

The growing trend toward respect for autonomy in health care was legislated in 1991 with the passage of the federal Patient Self Determination Act. As a result of this legislation, health care providers and health care institutions are mandated to give priority to the patient's treatment preferences, even when those preferences limit the use of treatments that will sustain life. Today, in the literature, respect for autonomy is considered the cornerstone of biomedical ethics in the United States.

The acceptance of the decision to stop aggressive treatment on a resident and concentrate on comfort care measures poses special difficulties for CNAs working in long term care settings. Among staff, CNAs typically spend the most time with individual residents and provide the bulk of hands-on care. Unlike acute care settings, nursing homes provide the unique experience of caring for the same individuals for months, years, and even decades. During this time nursing assistants often form close bonds with their residents. While there are a number of positive components to this aspect of nursing home life, this also contributes to the difficulties CNAs have in accepting the upcoming death of a resident. In itself, this intensive contact often leads to grief and sadness when a resident has died or is dying. Many CNAs who took part in this study expressed feelings of closeness to residents and the experience of loss when a resident died.

Added difficulties arise when a CNA is caring for a resident who has chosen not to continue life-sustaining medical treatment. As health care workers, CNAs have been trained to promote life, and may feel that accepting the decision to focus on comfort care measures and terminate aggressive treatment conflicts with their training and responsibilities. Additionally, after the decision to end aggressive treatment has been made, it is the nursing assistant who is expected to provide the hands-on care for the resident, at a time when even families sometimes pull away. When caring for a resident after life-sustaining treatment has been ended, CNAs may feel that they are contributing to the resident's death. This may increase the difficulty of working with the dying resident as well as lead to a decrease in feelings of well-being and job satisfaction.

The fact that nursing assistants are a fundamental component of resident care and crucial to the day-to-day functioning of the nursing home is obvious. However, despite this fact, the educational and emotional needs of nursing assistants have often been ignored. Nursing assistants are expected to provide hands-on care for residents including bathing, toileting, dressing, positioning, and comforting them, ideally with competency and compassion. Nurses no longer have the luxury of spending prolonged periods of time with residents due to a variety of causes, including cuts in staff as well as an increased focus on state-regulated documentation. Thus, the role of nursing assistants has become even more important in recent years as well as more central to the well-being of the resident.

For these reasons, it is necessary to educate nursing assistants about the ethical issues surrounding end-of-life treatment decision-making. Knowledge about issues such as advance directives, the importance of respecting autonomy, and the continued need for comfort care regardless of treatment decisions will provide nursing assistants with a structure in which to work and a greater understanding of the decision-making process. Moreover, providing nursing assistants with the opportunity and forum to discuss their feelings and attitudes about these issues may help them cope psychologically and emotionally with difficult cases that arise. It is important for nursing assistants to know that their contributions are important and necessary and their opinions and feelings are respected. Nursing assistants fulfill a crucial role within the nursing home environment. It is our obligation to recognize their needs and try to meet them. It is hoped that providing education and support for nursing assistants will also in turn lead to improved care for the elderly resident.

3

Structure of the Program and General Recommendations

This program was designed to educate CNAs and to provide a forum to discuss the difficult ethical issues related to end-of-life decision-making. Throughout the project we emphasize three central points: autonomy of the resident, the importance of comfort care at the end of life, and the role of the CNA. Additional topics covered include: advance directives, truth-telling, staff-interactions, family decision-making, comfort care, spirituality in the nursing home, and barriers to service.

WHAT YOU WILL FIND IN THIS WORKBOOK

As noted earlier, this workbook is designed to enable individual nursing homes to conduct the ethics education program on their own. The workbook is arranged in the following fashion: practical program advice, a description of the questionnaire session, an overview of the educational sessions, and a detailed delineation of the educational sessions focusing on the specific areas highlighted in the project. Throughout the educational sessions, the workbook refers to questions in the questionnaire, and discusses how the CNAs in the original study responded to them. There are periodic "Discussion Tips" that give guidance to the instructor in methods of fostering more verbal interaction among the CNAs, as well as "Prompt Questions" that may be used to elicit from the participating CNAs how they feel about certain issues. There is also "Educational Information" about specific topics included throughout, as well as the findings from the original study. For many of the topics, there are also "Practical Policy Implications" for the nursing home that suggest helpful mechanisms the facility may wish to adopt.

At the back of the workbook, there are numerous appendices. Included among them are the questionnaire, a blank ethics education instructional booklet, an ethics education booklet containing the responses from the original study, and an evaluation form. There are also blank health care proxy and living will forms that are typical of New York State forms, but will give participants an idea of what such forms look like. And finally, there is an abbreviated version of this workbook (called the CNA ethics booklet) that can be duplicated and distributed to CNAs participating in the program.

PRACTICAL PROGRAM ADVICE

We recommend the program be divided into four sessions with an optional fifth session. The purpose of the first session is to examine nursing assistants' current knowledge about end-of-life ethics and their attitudes towards these issues. In this session CNAs are asked to complete the Ethics Questionnaire. The information that is obtained from the initial session is then used as a starting point for the three educational/discussion sessions that follow. A minimum of one hour is needed for each session. This will allow time to discuss the topics in detail. In a fifth session the Ethics Questionnaire can be re-administered to assess whether there have been any changes in CNAs' knowledge and attitudes.

As many CNAs as desired can take part in the first and fifth sessions. However, during the three educational sessions it is best to break up into groups of five to ten CNAs. While this number can obviously be varied according to the needs of the nursing home, we have found this to be the optimal number for a good discussion group, though we have run sessions with as few as three CNAs and as many as twenty.

In order to facilitate open discussions among nursing assistants, it is preferable not to have anyone with direct authority over the nursing assistants present during the sessions. The confidentiality of the questionnaires and of any comments made during the sessions should be stressed. The nursing assistants should be instructed not to write their names on the questionnaires and assured that everything said during the educational sessions will be kept confidential. While the feelings of the CNAs may be discussed as a whole it should be emphasized that no one's individual responses will be identified.

The nature of this program is not to provide answers to the difficult and complex ethical dilemmas which arise at the end of life. Often clear-cut answers can not be provided and the best solutions will likely differ from case to case and from facility to facility (as many of the CNAs with whom we worked pointed out). What this program does do is open discussion about difficult issues. It provides the opportunity to express one's own feelings about end-of-life treatment, and allows participants to hear other points of view.

Other than the questions on the first two pages of the questionnaire, most do not have right or wrong answers. The questions are designed to examine people's beliefs and attitudes towards difficult issues. The opportunity to hear others talk about their different perspectives is an important part of the program. It allows people to realize that others may have different opinions and beliefs than their own and that there may be legitimate reasons behind these different opinions. It also highlights the complexity of the ethical issues when more than one perspective is presented. Hopefully, the acceptance of different opinions within the group discussion will generalize to an appreciation of the point that residents and families also have a wide range of feelings towards these same issues. It is worthwhile to point this out every once in a while during the discussion sessions: "Just as there are differences of opinions right here in this room over this issue, residents, family members, and other staff can also have a wide range of feelings based upon their own experiences and beliefs."

THE PROGRAM SESSIONS

4

Session 1: Questionnaire Session

In the questionnaire session the nursing assistants should be presented with a brief overview of the project and then given the Ethics Questionnaire to complete (located in Appendix A). This session will take between 45 minutes and one hour.

1. OVERVIEW

- Provide the CNAs with a brief introduction to the program. Tell them what the program is about and what topics will be covered. An introduction to the program can be found on pages 1–3 in "The CNA's Ethics Booklet" (Appendix F). You may choose to go through these pages with the CNAs and use this as the introduction to the program.
- Tell the CNAs the timetable of the program. For example: "This is the first session of the program. In this session you will fill out a questionnaire examining what you think and feel about different things like patient autonomy and advance directives. After this there will be three one-hour educational/discussion sessions, during which these issues will be discussed in more detail." Give the CNAs a handout with the dates of the future sessions so they know in advance when all of the sessions will be held.

2. ADMINISTERING THE QUESTIONNAIRE

- Hand out copies of the questionnaire (found in Appendix A).

We have found that the best way to administer the questionnaire is to read each question aloud as the nursing assistants follow along in their own copies. (Some CNAs may prefer to complete the questionnaire on their own, which is also fine). Although the questionnaire has been rated at an eighth grade reading level, some of the questions may need clarification. Reading the questions aloud will help to ensure that the questions are understandable. It will also facilitate questions if anything is unclear. Additionally, we have found that CNAs often find the questions more interesting when they are read aloud.

Model Instructions That Can Be Used When Administering the Questionnaire

"In this session there is a long questionnaire for you to fill out. It asks about how you feel about a lot of different end-of-life issues like living wills and health care proxies, care of dying residents, and patient autonomy. In the next few sessions we will have the chance to talk about these issues in much more detail.

"Do not put your name on the questionnaires. We want to know as a group what you think and feel about these issues; we don't need to know how each of you feels individually.

"Only the questions on the first couple of pages have right or wrong answers. If you are not sure what the correct answer is don't worry about it—most people do not know the answers to these questions. If you know what the answer is, circle the correct answer. If you are not sure what the correct answer is, you can either give it your best guess or circle "don't know." The rest of the questions are asking for your opinions; what you think about these issues. Your opinions may be different from the people you are sitting next to or from mine and that's fine; there are no right or wrong answers.

"We'll go through the questionnaire together and I'll read it out loud. Please stop me if you have any questions. Let me know if I'm reading it too quickly or too slowly."

Additional Instructions

If the CNAs say that the questions are hard to answer, they aren't sure how they feel, or that sometimes they "agree" and sometimes they "disagree," reassure them that they are right; these *are* difficult questions to answer, especially with words like "agree" and "disagree." Tell them to answer as best they can and during the discussion session the issues can be discussed in a lot more detail. Let them know that part of the purpose of the questions is for them to start thinking about some of the issues that will be discussed during the educational discussion sessions.

Some of the CNAs may want to write down the reasoning for some of their answers or they may want to qualify their answers with a "sometimes" or "it depends"; let them do this if they want to, but continue to go through the questionnaire at a reasonable pace so that you can finish within the allotted time.

5

Sessions 2–4: Educational Sessions/Overview

The next three sessions are educational/discussion sessions. The questions that were on the ethics questionnaire are used as the basis for discussion and teaching. The following is a general outline for the educational sessions, but you should feel free to go at your own pace and cover the topics in a different order.

A. OUTLINE

Educational Session 1

- Advance Directives

    1) Health Care Proxies
    2) Living Wills

- The Family and the Doctor in the Decision-Making Process
- Support for Families and Staff

Educational Session 2

- Comfort Issues
- Autonomy and Treatment
- Truth-Telling

Educational Session 3

- Barriers to Care
- Financial Concerns
- The CNA as Part of the Health Care Team
- CNA Comfort with Caring for Residents who are not Receiving Curative Treatment
- Summary of Program Highlights

B. PREPARATION FOR THE EDUCATIONAL SESSIONS

1. After the CNAs complete the Ethics Questionnaire in the first session, calculate the percentages of CNAs that gave each possible answer (e.g., 30% answered "AGREE,"

50% answered "DISAGREE," 10% answered "DON'T KNOW," and 10% did not answer the question).

2. Fill in the percentages for each question in the blank educational instruction booklet located in Appendix B. Include the percentage of subjects who did not answer the question with those who answered "DON'T KNOW."

3. Make copies of the completed educational instruction booklet for yourself and each of the CNAs. This will be the focus of the three educational sessions. The workbook is set up to help facilitate discussion as you proceed through the educational instruction booklet. The questions in the workbook are covered in the same order as they are in the booklet.

C.   DISCUSSION SESSION TIPS

The discussion sessions have a free-flow format based on the responses to the ethics questionnaire. Different issues will arise depending on the different experiences of the CNAs (both personal and professional) as well as the dynamics of the group. To facilitate discussion we suggest any and all of the following practices:

- Go over each of the questions on the Ethics Questionnaire and the CNAs' responses to them. For example, say to the CNAs: "The next question is-It is possible to prevent a dying resident from feeling much pain—70% percent of you agreed with that question, 20% of you disagreed, and about 10% of you weren't sure how you felt. What do you think? How did you answer the question? Why do you feel that way?"
- Discuss the educational information that is provided in the various sections throughout the workbook.
- Use the prompt questions and case scenarios. We include a list of prompt questions throughout the workbook to help facilitate discussions. There are also a number of cases provided for discussion.
- Discuss cases from your own experience or cases that have come up in the facility and ask the CNAs to give their opinions about these cases.
- Often, without prompting, CNAs will choose to share their experiences with death, dying, and treatment decision-making both from their professional and personal lives. It adds a great deal to the group discussion when CNAs discuss their personal experiences and how they were affected by them.
- Discuss the original study findings that are listed in each section. Throughout the workbook the CNAs' responses and attitudes from the original study are presented. (The overall study responses to the questions on the Ethics Questionnaire are listed in Appendix C.) Are the findings in your facility the same or different than the overall findings from the twenty-eight nursing homes that took part in the study? Discuss with the CNAs at your facility how the CNAs at the other facilities felt about these issues and ask whether they feel the same way. What do the CNAs think about the similarities and differences between your facility and the overall findings from the original study? What do they think might be the cause of any dramatic differences that are found? (Keep in mind that the results reported in Appendix C reflect the combined responses from all of the nursing homes. They do not indicate the wide variability found among the individual nursing homes.)

6

Educational Sessions

ADVANCE DIRECTIVES

QUESTIONS 1–12

Give each of the CNAs a copy of a health care proxy form and a copy of a living will. You can use those found in Appendix E of the workbook, however, these are New York State forms and you will likely wish to use forms from your own state.

Discussion Tips

When explaining health care proxies and living wills it is useful to discuss how they are beneficial for everyone, not just the residents. Discuss how the CNAs can use advance directives in their own lives. This allows the CNAs to identify with these issues.

Educational Information

Health Care Proxy (Also Called the Durable Power of Attorney for Health Care)

What is a health care proxy?
   A *health care proxy* is a document in which you state who you would want to make decisions for you if there ever came a time when you could no longer make decisions on your own. The health care proxy is a legal document in most states.
   The person you name to make decisions for you in your health care proxy is called your *health care agent.* Your health care agent is only asked to make health care decisions for you if you no longer have decision-making ability.
   A health care proxy can always be changed. As long as you can make decisions, you can change the instructions in your health care proxy. You can just rip up your old health care proxy and make a new one. If you have more than one health care proxy your most recently dated one will be followed.
   The purpose of the health care proxy is to try to ensure that your treatment wishes are carried out even when you can no longer communicate those wishes to the health care team.

Completing the Health Care Proxy Form

Some of the CNAs may want to take home copies of the health care proxy form either for themselves or for someone in their families. Therefore it is useful to go through the document and review how to

135

fill it out. Additionally, explaining how to complete the form again personalizes the issue of advance directives and starts to get the CNAs thinking about what they would want in these situations. This helps them identify with residents, their families, and the difficult issues with which they are faced.

It is important to point out that the health care proxy form is a very simple form to complete and despite the fact that it is a legal document, in most states there is no need for a lawyer. It is an extremely accessible form for everyone.

The health care proxy must be completed by you while you have the ability to make decisions. If the form is filled out when you can no longer make decisions it is invalid. Therefore, in the nursing home for example, the health care proxy must be completed while the resident is able to choose a health care agent. The family can not designate a health care agent for the resident. It should be recognized, however, that residents often have the ability to pick who they want to make treatment decisions for them even after they have lost the ability to make more complex decisions.

The person you choose as your health care agent should be someone you trust to carry out your wishes. The decisions health care agents are faced with are literally ones of life and death and are often difficult to carry out (for example stopping a feeding tube even when knowing the individual would not want it). If *you* complete a health care proxy form it is important for you to discuss end-of-life treatment wishes with your health care agent so that your agent will be able to make the decisions you would want. Additionally, if *you are chosen as someone else's health care agent* it is important for you to ask that person about his or her treatment wishes. What sometimes happens is that the health care agent does not know she has been designated as the agent until she is contacted to make a decision. By this point the patient or resident is no longer able to express his wishes.

What Is a Living Will?

A living will is a document made out by you stating your treatment wishes, to be followed if you can no longer make decisions or are unable to communicate. In many states it is a legal document and/or it is often accepted as evidence of an individual's treatment wishes. Like the health care proxy, your living will can always be updated and revised as long as you still have decision-making abilities.

Hospitals and nursing homes have a legal obligation to abide by a patient's or a resident's advance directives.

You should tell people you are close to (especially your health care agent) that you have completed a health care proxy and/or living will. You should also either give one or two people a copy of the forms or tell them where they can easily find them (a safe deposit box is not a good place to keep these forms since it is not easily accessible) in case the forms are ever needed.

Study Findings[1]

Generally, CNAs were more familiar with living wills than with health care proxies. Participants often believed that health care agents' decision-making powers are more extensive

---

[1]All reported study findings are from the original Greenwall study. See page 123.

than they really are. About a third of CNAs (34%) incorrectly stated that the health care agent could sell the resident's home and over half (54%) stated the health care agent could make financial decisions for the residents. On the other hand, more than 50 percent of the CNAs correctly responded that health care agents could make a variety of treatment decisions for residents, the most (60%) stating that "yes" the health care agent could tell the doctor not to start a feeding tube.

In contrast, with respect to living wills, most of the CNAs correctly stated that doctors could not amputate (79%) or put in a feeding tube (83%) if the resident had a living will stating that he/she would not want it.

Practical Implications for the Nursing Home

In many facilities, CNAs are excluded from discussions of the overall treatment plan and are not told about the existence of advance directives. This may result in increased difficulty when a decision is made to stop life-sustaining treatment. During the project a number of CNAs stated that they feel better if they know the treatment course carried out is what *the resident* would want. It is helpful for staff to know that the resident had previously specified these wishes and/or that the person making decisions (if it is not the resident) was chosen by the resident. If CNAs do not know about the existence of a health care proxy or a living will they do not have the reassurance that they are acting according to the wishes of the resident. Moreover, the discontinuation of treatment may lead CNAs to question the motives of the family and other staff members as well as feel guilty about their own participation in treatment.

CNAs also stated they would prefer to know as soon as possible that a resident has a health care proxy or living will so that they are psychologically prepared if there is a decision to end aggressive medical treatment.

THE FAMILY AND THE DOCTOR IN THE DECISION-MAKING PROCESS

The next series of questions examine CNAs' opinions about who should make treatment decisions for residents who can no longer make decisions on their own.

QUESTIONS 48, 49, 50, 30, 31, 51

Prompt Questions

- Who do you think is best able to make treatment decisions for the resident?
- Why do you think the family should or should not be able to make these decisions?
- Why do you think the doctor should or should not be able to make these decisions?
- Who would you want to make health care decisions for you?
- Who would you want to make decisions for your mother or father if they could not make health care decisions for themselves?
- Should a family member who rarely visits be able to make health care decisions for the resident?

- Do you think a family member can live far away but still care about their relative in a nursing home?

Study Findings

Most CNAs (82%) believed families should be able to make treatment decisions, when the resident can no longer make those decisions, even if there are no advance directives. When asked whether the doctor, the family, or someone else should make decisions for mentally impaired residents, 42% said the family, 32% said the doctor and 18% indicated the family and the doctor should work together to make decisions.

CNAs who chose the "family" generally said that "families know the residents longer and better than anyone else and therefore are most qualified to make these types of decisions." They often said if they were in a similar situation they would want their families to make health care decisions for them and they would want to be the ones making decisions for their family members. These CNAs said doctors have usually only known the resident for a short time and do not know the resident's individual history, values, or religious beliefs. One CNA said she felt that "doctors in nursing homes see all of the residents as little old ladies with little to differentiate one from the other."

Despite the fact that many CNAs thought families should be able to make decisions, they were uncomfortable with the thought of family members making treatment decisions if they were not perceived as actively involved (e.g., did not visit regularly) or did not have a good relationship with the resident. Thus, although most CNAs felt families should be able to make treatment decisions for their relatives, it was somewhat dependent on their perception of the relationship between the family member and the resident.

CNAs who said the doctor is the best person to make treatment decisions for the resident generally gave the reason that the doctor is trained in these matters. "Doctors know about different treatment options and therefore will know what is best for the resident. Families are not medically trained and do not have the ability to make treatment decisions." These CNAs were concerned that families might be motivated by factors other than the best interest of the resident. For example, CNAs said, "Some families may be more concerned with their inheritance than the resident's well-being. The doctor has the resident's best interest at heart." At many facilities CNAs had stories about residents who they felt were neglected by family members. CNAs often said they did not know a resident had family until the resident was dying and the family came to claim the belongings. In these circumstances CNAs said they would feel more comfortable with the doctor or other staff members making treatment decisions.

A third group of CNAs said the family and doctor should work together to find the best possible option for the resident. "The doctor can provide the medical information while the family provides information about the lifestyle and values of the resident." Thus the family in consultation with the doctor may be able to best carry out the resident's wishes. Most of the CNAs in this category felt families should have the final say in the treatment decision.

Practical Policy Implications for the Nursing Home

We need to include CNAs in the ongoing process of the case. The CNAs are often exposed to only one perspective. A resident may in fact have a very concerned or involved family member but the CNA may not realize this because the family member visits during a different shift, or the family member may not be able to visit and rather calls the nurse or social worker on the unit. If the CNAs are aware of this they may feel better about treatment decisions made by family members. Similarly, other staff members may be concerned about a resident but the CNAs may not recognize this if they are not included in the team meetings or other discussions about the resident.

Additional Issues

It is important to keep cultural differences concerning the use of nursing homes in mind and to discuss this issue with the CNAs. CNAs often told us that in the countries they are from people would not place their family members in nursing homes; rather, the family would care for the older person at home. Moreover, if for some reason a person was placed in a hospital or nursing home, the family would be there constantly. As one CNA said, "In this country people don't have respect for their elderly, they throw them out when they get old." It is important to recognize these views about nursing homes and family involvement and discuss them openly.

Prompt Discussion

An interesting interaction between two CNAs that occurred at one of the nursing homes we visited illustrates this issue of cultural differences.

CNA 1: "In my country you would never put your parents in a nursing home."
CNA 2: "In my country you would never put your parents in a nursing home either, but I live here now and if I want to send my kids to university I have to work during the day. I can't afford to stay home and take care of my parents. I have to work."

- Ask the CNAs to give their opinions about this conversation and ask how they feel overall about placing a family member in a nursing home.

QUESTION 51 EXAMINES WHETHER FAMILIES SHOULD BE ABLE TO OVERRULE RESIDENTS WHO CAN MAKE DECISIONS IF RESIDENTS ARE REFUSING TREATMENT

Prompt Questions

- Who should we listen to: the resident or the family?
- Let's say you have a 95 year-old man who says, "I'm old and tired; I don't want the antibiotics," and the family says, "Just give it to him; put it in his apple sauce he will never know the difference"; what should you do?
- Do you feel it is different to accept a resident's decision not to take antibiotics (a painless short-term treatment) versus a decision not to continue something like dialysis (a much more intrusive, long term treatment)?

Study Findings

The majority of CNAs said families should not be able to overrule residents who can still make decisions (65%). They said residents' autonomy should be respected even if they choose not to have life-sustaining treatment. They stated that the primary concern and responsibility of the nursing home staff should be to the resident, not the resident's family. "Unless you are in the resident's shoes you do not know what he's feeling and you should respect his wishes."

CNAs who answered "yes," the family should be able to overrule the resident, often spoke about the situation in personal terms. They said, "Look, if it were my parents I would want them to get treatment, even if they didn't want it and I would ask the doctor to treat them or I would tell my parents that they had to get treatment."

Discussion Tips

Ask the CNAs what they think about the above response "if it were my parent I would make sure they got treatment." Point out to the CNAs that this response highlights the difficulty of end-of-life decision-making. While legally there is a responsibility to abide by the patient's wishes it is not always an easy thing for staff to do or families to live with. It is important to emphasize that there are situations when residents make a treatment choice that we may not want them to make or that we may not have chosen for them or ourselves, but legally it is their right to make the decision. At the same time we have to recognize that situations like these may be difficult for family and staff and that they need to be supported at these times.

Additionally, the family does have the right to tell the resident about their own feelings and why they personally want the resident to receive treatment. The facility, on the other hand, has a legal responsibility to find out what the resident's needs and wishes are and to place these as the priority.

SUPPORT FOR FAMILIES AND STAFF

QUESTIONS 13A, 13B, 13C—RESIDENT AND FAMILY SUPPORT IN TREATMENT DECISION-MAKING

Study Findings

CNAs were generally positive in feeling that at their facilities, staff try to find out the types of treatment residents want, tell residents about their treatment options, and help residents and their families to make treatment choices.

QUESTION 13D—FAMILY SUPPORT

Prompt Questions

- Do you feel families get emotional support here?
- If you feel families get support, who do you think they get it from?
- What types of things are done or can be done to give support to families?

Study Findings

About half the CNAs felt that families of dying residents always get support and almost another quarter of the CNAs said families get support at least some of the time. When asked "who gives support to families" CNAs often said they are the ones who give the most support to families. They felt this support was expressed mainly by listening to the families, and spending time with them and the residents.

In addition to themselves, others who were mentioned as giving support to families varied from facility to facility but included nurses, social workers, and clergy.

QUESTION 13E—STAFF SUPPORT

CNAs often have strong feelings about this question. Many feel that they do not get support or recognition for the hard work they do. It is important to encourage discussion about practical ways to provide support for CNAs. It may not be possible to increase staff (a suggestion that is often made), however, it may be possible to allow CNAs to go to the funerals of residents they care for or to increase the amount of positive recognition given for a job well done.

Prompt Questions

- Do you feel close to the residents you take care of?
- Do you feel you need support or counseling when caring for dying residents or do you feel this is a part of your job that you just have to get used to?
- Have you ever had a case which you found particularly difficult? What was it?
- Is there someone you can talk to about difficult cases?
- Do you think it would be helpful to have ongoing supportive programs?
- What do you feel would help you if a resident you felt close to passed away?
- How do you take care of yourself when you have a stressful day on the job?

Study Findings

Overall, 42% of CNAs said they "never" get emotional support or counseling when caring for dying residents. However, responses varied substantially across nursing homes.

During the discussion sessions CNAs stated that not enough attention is paid to their emotional needs when caring for residents who are dying. Many said there is an understanding, whether spoken or unspoken, that they are not supposed to get too close to residents. The implication being that if they don't allow themselves to become attached to residents they won't become upset when a resident becomes ill or dies.

Case Example

One CNA said that the first time one of her residents died it was about a year after she started working. She was very upset when this happened and started to cry. The nurse on her unit called her into her office and said, "You don't have to cry about this," and then she sent her to clean the body. The nurse wasn't trying to be hurtful. However, the CNA felt the nurse didn't acknowledge her grief when the resident died. She said, "It's like you aren't allowed to be sad when a resident dies. It's just supposed to be part of the job."

A few CNAs we encountered stated they do not get close to residents. Rather, they said they provide the same good quality care to everyone without forming close attachments. Most CNAs, however, felt this was not a realistic expectation. Additionally, many said they can provide better care by developing relationships with the residents, knowing more about them, and being able to treat the residents as individuals. Almost all the CNAs admitted to having favorite residents with whom they have special relationships.

Most CNAs said the emotional support they receive comes from other CNAs. There is a strong feeling that they understand and help each other through difficult situations. Many also expressed the feeling that the professional staff does not appreciate the difficulty of their job.

This is not to say CNAs at all nursing homes felt they did not get support from other staff members. Often there was a particular person in nursing or staff development, and in a couple of instances social work, whom CNAs felt they could go to for support. There were also a few facilities at which CNAs said they get support from both fellow CNAs and the nurses on their units. These CNAs said the nurses they work with also get very attached to the residents. One CNA said, "Sometimes you'll walk into the room of a dying resident and the nurse will be on one side of the bed stroking the resident's hand and the CNA will be on the other side."

CNAs generally did not feel they needed constant support on the job. Rather, they indicated that certain cases are more difficult than others and that is the time when support would be most appreciated.

Discussion Tips

Ask the CNAs to discuss the factors they find most difficult about working with dying residents. Next, ask them what types of things would help them in their work. Below is a list of things that the CNAs who took part in the original study found to be most difficult on the job as well as a list of things they identified as helpful.

Situations that CNAs Described as Most Difficult

- When a resident the CNA is close to becomes very sick and/or dies.
- Difficult work situations (e.g., caring for a resident with gangrene who refuses to have an amputation).
- Not knowing whether it is the resident's wishes or the family's wishes that are being carried out (e.g., has a feeding tube been stopped because it is what the resident would want or has it been stopped because the family wants it to stop).
- When the CNA first starts to work in the nursing home and in particular the first time one of the CNA's residents dies.
- When a resident dies while the CNA is taking care of the resident or has just finished taking care of the resident (e.g., feeding or bathing the resident). CNAs sometimes feel they might have done something wrong and that's why the resident died.
- Caring for the resident's body after death.

Things CNAs Identified as Helpful

- Allowing CNAs to go to the funerals of residents they cared for or were close to and if needed providing the transportation for them to get to the services. CNAs feel this would be helpful both to themselves and to family members.
- Including CNAs in the overall care plan of the resident. This way they would have more information about the resident's condition and would know what to expect.
- Informing CNAs when the resident first comes on the unit whether or not the resident has an advance directive and what the resident's end-of-life wishes are. One CNA said that he felt very badly about a resident who was no longer receiving treatment. He later learned that the resident had a living will stating that this was his wish. The CNA said he then felt better about the situation.
- Telling CNAs about the treatments they provide. CNAs said they want to know more about different treatments. For example, if they are instructed to put a cream on a resident, they would like to know what the cream does.
- Providing a supportive environment to discuss difficult cases. At some facilities CNAs did have supportive discussion sessions with staff after particularly difficult cases. CNAs said this was helpful and they suggested having these types of sessions while cases are ongoing rather than only after the resident has died.
- Giving constructive advice. At one nursing home where support sessions were available CNAs said it would be helpful if the person directing the groups gave concrete advice rather than just asking how the CNAs felt about the case. (Concrete advice can include information about treatment, how to provide the resident with best possible comfort and spiritual care, and suggesting that the CNAs try to watch out for each other and be able to ask for and offer added help when necessary.)
- Providing CNAs with extra information about caring for the dying, including both the treatment component as well as the emotional and psychological issues involved. At some nursing homes CNAs said that hospice inservices they participated in were helpful.
- CNAs often talked about the difficulty of taking care of the resident's body after the resident has died. Some CNAs said the nurses on their units were helpful and gave them time to adjust before they had them clean a body themselves. These nurses often had them watch other CNAs a few times so that they would feel more comfortable.
- Increasing the amount of positive reinforcement given to CNAs for a job well done. CNAs repeatedly told us they always hear about the mistakes they make but it's rare for them to receive credit when they deserve it. When CNAs do receive positive recognition they are very proud of themselves and their work. For example one CNA told us, "I was named employee of the month, they really love me here; they know I do a good job." CNAs are very appreciative of any honors bestowed on them, even something as simple as a CNA day. CNAs said they would like people to say to them, "You are taking really good care of Mrs. X. She looks really good today."

Practical Policy Implications for the Nursing Home

Telling CNAs not to get close to residents sets up unrealistic expectations. Not only does it make CNAs more reluctant to seek out support it also makes them feel they are not doing their job properly. According to this ideal, CNAs should be able to provide good intensive hands-on care for people, often over years, without actually caring about them. Moreover, there has been a move towards *permanent* assignments of residents (as many CNAs put it "till death do us part") increasing the intensity of the relationship between resident and CNA.

Even if CNAs are not explicitly told not to get close to residents, they often think this is what is expected of them. At most of the facilities where we conducted the project, administration clearly recognized the importance of the CNAs, the difficulties of the CNAs' job, and the often close relationship between residents and CNAs. The CNAs, however, were rarely aware of this recognition held by the administration. Frank discussion concerning the difficulties of caring for dying residents and open recognition of the relationship between staff and residents may alleviate some of the misunderstanding and miscommunication between CNAs and other staff members. It is not enough just to recognize that close relationships often exist between residents and CNAs (as well as other staff members). We have to begin providing formal and informal support systems for staff on an ongoing basis.

One of the most basic areas to improve CNA support is to consciously increase the amount of positive reinforcement given to CNAs for providing good care to residents. As one CNA stated, having someone say "you are doing a good job" or "thank you" can be more important than a financial bonus.

COMFORT ISSUES

The following section focuses on the comfort of dying residents. It should be stressed to the CNAs that for many nursing home residents compassionate comfort care is just as important, if not more important, than aggressive medical treatment and that they (the CNAs) are the ones who provide the essentials of hands-on comfort care.

Educational Information

Barriers to Comfort Care

Solomon and colleagues (1993) found that out of 687 physicians and nurses from five hospitals, 87% believed that "it is possible to prevent dying residents from feeling much pain." On the other hand, 81% reported that the most common form of narcotic abuse is the *undertreatment* of pain. This indicates that while health care professionals believe we have the ability to alleviate the pain of the dying, this outcome is frequently not achieved.

There are a number of factors which may act as barriers to the delivery of adequate pain relief:

- Fear of hastening death. Solomon et al. (1993) found that 44% of nurses and 33% of doctors believe the delivery of inadequate pain medication is due to clinician's fears that increasing the amount of medication will hasten the patient's death.
- Fear of the patient or resident becoming addicted to the pain medication (Wilson & Daley, 1998; The Hastings Center, 1987).
- Belief that the patient does not really need the medication.

- Health care professionals lack of knowledge concerning the appropriate use of drugs and dosages to relieve pain (The Hastings Center, 1987).
- Inadequate attention paid to signs of discomfort. This is particularly important for residents with dementia. A study by Morrison and Siu (1998) found that patients who were unable to communicate received significantly less pain medication than residents who could communicate and had similar diagnoses.
- Patients' reluctance to increase their pain medication due to misinformation about either their pain or their medication.
- Patients' reluctance to "bother" the health care staff about their pain.
- Misunderstanding of patient directives. A resident who is requesting not to continue life-sustaining treatment is not asking for an end to all treatment. The resident still needs and wants comfort care. In fact, when the resident is dying he/she is especially in need of comfort care.
- Fear of being with a dying resident. Many people fear death and it can be difficult for people, even health care workers who frequently come into contact with the dying, to be alone in a room with someone who is near death.

As with all types of treatments, individual choices concerning the treatment of pain will vary across individuals. Some people's primary concern is to alleviate any discomfort or pain even if sedation is necessary, while others value the continuation of treatment, and others desire quality time with friends and family. A primary function of the health care team is to determine the residents' wishes and ensure to the best of their abilities that those wishes are carried out.

The CNA's Role in Comfort Care

While appropriate medication is often supplied for pain relief, it is important to emphasize that there is a wide range of comfort measures which can be provided by CNAs. These include:

- Positioning—At its most basic, positioning is needed for good circulation and to prevent skin breakdown. However, positioning also includes subtle aspects of care such as knowing certain residents like to face a particular direction, or want their favorite blanket or pillow next to them, or want to sit exactly five and a half feet from the nurses' station. These are the things that differentiate each resident from his/her neighbor and are opportunities to show respect for the resident's individual needs.
- Hygiene—It is a given that residents should always be kept clean as well as comfortable. As is the case with positioning, extra touches can be provided for hygiene. In our facility some of the CNAs call this "beauty care." This includes: braiding the resident's hair, applying makeup, and generally caring for the outward appearance of the resident. This can make the resident feel better about him or herself and even if the resident is unaware of her/his appearance it increases the human contact between the CNA and the resident. It may also be comforting for families to see this kind of care given to the resident.
- Cold Compresses—Along with acetaminophen, cold compresses can be effectively used to reduce fever and soothe the resident.

- Mouth Care—Mouth care has been found to be an extremely important component of comfort care. While older residents who are dying often cannot tell us what makes them uncomfortable, studies have been done with cancer patients to determine sources of discomfort. Cancer patients who were no longer taking food or water by mouth or by feeding tube/IV reported that discomfort due to thirst or dry mouth could be alleviated with the use of ice chips or swabs (McCann, Hall, & Groth-Juncker, 1994). Dry mouth can be a source of extreme discomfort but it is one that can be remedied relatively easily.
- Touch—Just touching the resident's hand or brushing the resident's hair lets the resident know that there is someone nearby who cares.
- Talking to the Residents—Many residents have few visitors and are very lonely. Having someone pay attention and talk to them can be soothing to residents. Even if the resident can no longer understand and respond, the sound of a familiar voice still gives comfort.
- Paying Attention to Resident's Condition—CNAs spend more time with residents than any other member of the health care team. As a result they are more likely to sense a change in the comfort level of the resident. CNAs should feel they can express their concerns about resident comfort to the unit nurses and that their opinions are valued.

QUESTIONS 37, 19, 20A, AND 20B EXAMINE WHETHER CNAS FEEL SOME OF THE TREATMENTS GIVEN TO DYING RESIDENTS ARE TOO UNCOMFORTABLE FOR THEM

Prompt Questions

- Do you feel there are treatments that are too uncomfortable for residents?
- Do you feel you can tell when one of your residents is uncomfortable?
- Can you tell when a resident is uncomfortable even when they can't talk to you?

Study Findings

Question 37—CNAs were split about whether they feel some treatments we give residents are too uncomfortable for them. Forty-four percent of CNAs "disagreed" with this statement while 40% "agreed." During discussion sessions CNAs generally said residents are relatively comfortable. They also typically stated that if a treatment is uncomfortable but necessary for the health of the resident it should be carried out unless the resident is clearly dying, in which case the focus should be comfort rather than treatment. On the other hand, some CNAs felt that even when a resident is dying, life-prolonging treatment should be continued because no one knows for sure when the person is going to die. CNAs described many instances in which residents were expected to die and then lived for years.

Treatments that were mentioned as being uncomfortable for residents included:

- Straightening contracted limbs
- Feeding tubes
- Foley catheters
- Sitting residents up when they have bedsores

- Cleaning bedsores
- "Walking" residents when in actuality it is more like dragging residents
- Getting a resident out of bed every morning when the resident just wants to stay in bed. CNAs said once in a while they would like to be able to let a resident stay in bed if that is what the resident wants, particularly if the resident is dying or if the resident rarely makes this request.

A number of CNAs said they are reluctant to tell the nurse that a resident would be more comfortable without a certain treatment because they feel the nurse will think their motivation is laziness rather than resident comfort.

Case Example

One CNA said: "A while ago I was taking care of a very frail old lady who was dying. The nurse told me to give the lady a bath in the whirlpool. She was so frail though and I thought she should have a sponge bath instead. She couldn't even hold her head up on her own. I ended up giving her a bath in the whirlpool because the nurse told me to. The resident was scared to death in the bath. She only lived another few days. I think they should have let me give her a sponge bath. It was clear she was dying and we should have tried to just keep her comfortable and peaceful. The nurse might have thought I wanted to give her a sponge bath because it's easier but I just thought it would be better for the resident."

Study Findings

Questions 19, 20a, and 20b—(In the original study questions 20a and 20b were combined into one question: "Sometimes we make dying residents more uncomfortable by giving them tube feedings and IVs.") We originally expected that CNAs would report feeding tubes are more uncomfortable for residents than being fed by mouth. Surprisingly, 56% of CNAs "agreed" we sometimes make dying residents more uncomfortable by continuing to give them food and water by mouth while slightly fewer (42%) "agreed" we sometimes make dying residents more uncomfortable by feeding them with feeding tubes. During the discussion sessions CNAs stated they often feel they are forcing residents to eat when they feed them by mouth. They said it can be very frustrating when the nurses tell them they have to get more food into the residents and the residents don't cooperate with them. A number of CNAs said they think the residents just don't want to eat anymore and we shouldn't force them.

CNAs' feelings towards feeding tubes varied widely across facilities. The percentage of CNAs who "agreed" that sometimes we make dying residents more uncomfortable by giving them feeding tubes and IVs at each of the individual nursing homes ranged from 0% to 76%. Many CNAs felt that residents were adequately comfortable with feeding tubes and they believed the feeding tubes were necessary because they were keeping the residents alive. One CNA talked about a case in which a resident initially needed a feeding tube to stay alive and then made a full recovery and no longer required the tube feeding. In this case the resident would have died without the tube feeding, however, with it she recovered. Other CNAs greatly disliked feeding tubes and stated they would never want one for themselves or their family members. They said there is no quality of life for the person on the feeding tube. These CNAs viewed feeding tubes as prolonging death rather than life.

Discussion Tips

The reason for asking these questions is to raise sensitivity to resident discomfort. Nursing homes have been criticized for not paying enough attention to patient/resident discomfort, pain, and anxiety. Even if a particular treatment is necessary we should still be aware of any discomfort it causes and try to the best of our abilities to soothe and comfort the resident. Often the CNAs are in the best position to do this. Thus, the discussion throughout this section should emphasize causes of discomfort, ways of determining discomfort, and ways to alleviate discomfort. The fact that residents, particularly those with dementing illnesses, often cannot make their discomfort known should be stressed.

QUESTION 26 FOCUSES ON THE DELIVERY OF COMFORT CARE TO DYING RESIDENTS

Prompt Question

- What are some of the things that in your experience you have found help to make dying residents more comfortable?

Study Findings

The majority (63%) of CNAs "agreed" that it is possible to prevent dying residents from feeling much pain. During the discussion sessions CNAs initially spoke about the use of medication to relieve pain but then eventually began to discuss measures that they provide to increase comfort such as cold compresses, positioning, hand-holding, and in particular good mouth care.

Discussion Tips

Sometimes CNAs will discuss cases in which they were able to provide comfort to residents. CNAs greatly appreciate receiving positive reinforcement when they talk about these types of cases. Tell them that they did something beautiful and important for the resident. Comfort care is a crucial aspect of the CNA's job and one that CNAs should feel especially proud about being able to provide.

The following are case examples of comfort care from some of the CNAs who took part in the original Greenwall study (you may want to use these cases for discussion):

Case Examples

- At one nursing home we visited, staff place a particularly strong emphasis on comfort care. As a result, CNAs and nurses try to make sure that residents who are dying always have someone in the room with them. One night, this nursing home was short-staffed and there was nobody to sit with a resident who was dying. A CNA who was working on the night shift felt that someone needed to be in the room with the resident. This CNA had recently married and she called her husband, a construction worker, to come and stay with the resident. The husband came in and stayed with the resident all night.

- In another case a CNA told us that when she knew a resident who she was close to was dying, she went to her room and talked to her and held her hand. She said she was there for the resident at the end and she felt good about it and she thought it helped the resident.
- One CNA said that when a resident wants to go home she responds by saying, "Why do you want to do that? You have everything you need here. It's warm here, you have food here and we take care of you."
- Another CNA spoke about a resident she was caring for who had a living will that stated she would not want a feeding tube. The resident had experienced a stroke and could no longer swallow or communicate but she would sit up in her chair and her eyes would follow you around the room. The CNA said, "It was so sad; Mrs. L was so pretty. She would be happy to see me whenever I went to her room and she would give me a smile. Mrs. L used to love flowers so I always used to put a flower in a button-hole on her sweater to make her feel good."
- One CNA said she likes to be the person who wraps the bodies of her residents that pass away. She wants this opportunity to care for them until the end and she feels it gives her a sense of closure.

CNAs cannot spend indefinite periods of time providing comfort care to dying residents. They have too many other responsibilities and their workload is too large. During discussion they often said that they don't have the ability to spend as much time with the residents as each of the residents would like; they have too many other people to take care of. Ask the CNAs how they deal with these competing demands on their time and how they feel about it.

QUESTION 28 EXAMINES FEELINGS TOWARDS THE ADMINISTRATION OF PAIN MEDICATION

Study Findings

Just over half the CNAs (53%) "agreed" that sometimes it is right to give pain medication even if the person may die sooner, while 29% "disagreed" and 18% were not sure how they felt about it. A number of CNAs who agreed with this question said that if they were dying and in pain they would want the pain medication.

Educational Information

Clarify that this question examines the situation in which pain medication is given with the purpose of relieving pain. Although there may be a possibility that the pain medication will hasten death, this is not the intention or expectation of the treatment. This is considered acceptable both legally and medically. Question 31 is not asking about views towards physician-assisted suicide, in which case the doctor prescribes medication with the intention that the medication will cause the death of the resident. Physician-assisted suicide is a complex issue and at present not legally acceptable throughout the United States.

Historically, the permissibility of prescribing medication with the intention of relieving pain, even if a possible though not intended outcome is death, evolved from the principle of "double effect." The principle arose primarily out of the teachings of the Roman Catholic Church. A distinction is drawn between an intended outcome (e.g., giving enough pain medication with the intention of causing death) versus a non-intended though foreseeable outcome (e.g., giving pain medication with the intention of relieving pain with the knowledge that it is possible the pain medication will hasten a resident's death) (Beauchamp & Childress, 1989).

As with many treatments, individuals from different religious and cultural backgrounds, however, will have different views about the administration of pain medication, and these must be respected. Additionally, preferences towards pain medication will differ depending on the individual's current priorities. The primary concern of some people will be to relieve pain and discomfort while others will be more concerned with continuation of treatment or clarity of thought. It is very important for the health care team to try to determine the resident's wishes and carry them out to the best of their ability.

QUESTION 33 EXAMINES THE SPIRITUAL CARE OF DYING RESIDENTS

Prompt Questions

- What types of religious involvement are available to the residents here? What do you think of it?
- What does spiritual care mean to you?

Study Findings

A little over half the CNAs "disagreed" (54%) with the statement that "the spiritual needs of dying residents receive too little attention," while 30% "agreed" and 16% were not sure how they felt. During the discussion session it was apparent that most CNAs answered this question in relation to the availability and role of the clergy at their nursing home. Their views towards the involvement of clergy with the residents varied greatly from facility to facility. At some nursing homes staff said clergy were actively involved with residents and families and available both for formal services as well emotional support. At other facilities CNAs viewed clergy as primarily concerned with religious services but not the day-to-day needs of the residents.

Discussion Tips

One of the issues we discussed during the sessions was the different aspects of spiritual care which are available to the residents. CNAs initially spoke about the pastoral care in their facilities. However, spiritual care can also be conceptualized as any type of compassionate care that respects the religion and dignity of the person in life and in death. This includes sitting in the room with a dying resident, giving comfort to a resident who is scared, holding a resident's hand, and caring for the resident's body after death. Thus, in addition to the spiritual care provided by clergy, there is spiritual care which can be provided by all staff.

Case Example

During the educational sessions one of the CNAs told the following story: "I am Hindu and a little while ago I was taking care of an elderly Catholic lady who was dying. I bathed her and then I sat with her and said, "Look, I know you are suffering and you've suffered for a long time. If you want to go now, it's OK, I'm with you." The woman died soon thereafter.

As this story illustrates, one does not have to practice the same religion as another in order to provide spiritual care.

Case Example

While it is important to provide comfort, staff should be careful not to impose their own religious views on a resident—as sometimes happens:
"The other day we were walking by the room of a Jewish resident. The resident had Alzheimer's disease and was lying quietly in her bed and the radio in her room was tuned to a Christian talk show."

Ask the CNAs their opinions of the above two cases and ask them about their own experiences caring for dying residents.

QUESTIONS 17A, 17B, AND 18 EXAMINE HOW CNAS FEEL ABOUT GIVING FOOD AND WATER TO DYING RESIDENTS BY MOUTH AND BY FEEDING TUBE

Prompt Questions

- If a dying person asked you for food or water would you want to give it to them?
- Sometimes people talk about having learned while they were growing up to always offer food or water to someone who is very sick. Did any of you ever have this type of experience?

Study Findings

In the original study, questions 17a and 17b were combined into the single question: "A dying person should always be offered food and water by mouth." However, during the discussion sessions the CNAs often expressed the view that there should be two separate questions: one about water and one about food. Many felt that while you should always offer a dying person water, they were less sure about giving residents food.

A number of CNAs talked about the cultural importance of offering water to someone before they die. They often said that growing up it was stressed to them to give water to someone who is sick or dying as a way of providing comfort. Some CNAs spoke of their own experiences with dying family members. They often said that the dying person asked for water near death and they provided it for them (sometimes against the advice of other family members). They were typically thankful that they were able to provide this comfort to their family member.

CNAs said even if residents can't take very much liquid you should still give them a few drops of water to make sure their mouths and throats aren't dry. The CNAs talked about the importance of keeping residents' mouths and throats moist before they die so that they are not uncomfortable at the end.

One CNA said, "I know it sounds strange but if I am taking care of a resident and I don't have a chance to give them a drink of water and the resident dies my own throat feels dry. That's happened to me a couple of times. But if I do give them water I feel OK when they go."

Some CNAs had similar feelings towards offering food at the end of life. They generally felt that if a dying resident wants to eat they should be able to have what ever they want. They felt very positively about being able to provide whatever pleasure or comfort possible for dying residents. If the resident died shortly after having eaten, they were content in knowing they provided the resident with comfort and were fulfilling the resident's wishes. On the other hand, a number of CNAs said they are not comfortable when they have to feed a dying resident. They are scared that the resident will die while being fed or shortly afterwards and this actually happened in a number of cases. Unlike the CNAs discussed above (who were content in feeling that they delivered comfort to the resident by providing food shortly before death), these CNAs felt in some way guilty or responsible for the resident's death.

Discussion Tips

CNAs are very interested in discussing this question about whether or not food and water should be offered to dying residents. (During the study CNAs often asked if we could go to this question early on in the sessions.) This is likely because it is a practical issue and something they are faced with quite frequently. CNAs who feel we should give food and water to a dying resident like to talk about the positive comfort they can provide for dying residents. On the other hand, CNAs who are uncomfortable feeding dying residents can discuss their feelings and get feedback from the other CNAs. A few times during the original study, CNAs talked about feeling responsible for a resident's death because they fed the resident shortly before death.

Case Example

One CNA told the story that a nurse on her unit instructed her to feed a resident Ensure®. She fed the resident Ensure and the resident passed away. The CNA said at the time she felt very guilty and she still feels guilty about it. She said she had never talked to anybody about what happened. The other CNAs told her she shouldn't feel badly. The residents can die at anytime and all you can do is feed the person and take care of the person to the best of your ability. The discussion about this topic allowed the other CNAs to reassure her. She was also able to hear the perspective from some of the others that providing food at the end can be seen as comforting and positive.

QUESTION 18

Prompt Questions

- What if the person has a living will saying they wouldn't want a feeding tube?

Study Findings

The majority of CNAs (62%) agreed that "a dying person should always receive food and water, even by feeding tube if necessary." During discussion CNAs generally said the resident should get a feeding tube unless they gave instructions, in some fashion such as a living will, stating that they would not want it.

Practical Policy Implications for the Nursing Home

While CNAs often have opinions about the comfort of the resident they are typically left out of the treatment discussion in many facilities. Due to the close contact between CNAs and residents they may have important insights into those things which provide comfort or discomfort to the resident. We may lose important information about the resident if the CNA is excluded from care planning. Additionally, if the CNA is apprehensive about certain necessary treatments because they cause the resident discomfort, it is important to discuss with the CNA what the treatment is and why it is needed.

Another important issue is comfort care education. One of the things that CNAs told us they would like to receive more inservices on was appropriate comfort care for the dying. CNAs need to learn more about the positive things they can do for dying residents, particularly when aggressive medical treatment has been stopped. Education about the constructive steps that can be taken for the dying may alleviate some of the fear and stressors normally associated it. Additionally, positive reinforcement should be given to CNAs for providing good comfort care.

AUTONOMY AND TREATMENT

The next set of questions, 40, 41, 15, 16, (42, 43), 24, 27, and 22, examines CNAs' feelings concerning residents' rights to refuse life-sustaining treatment.

Educational Information

The Patient Self Determination Act (1991) requires all hospitals and nursing homes that receive Medicare and/or Medicaid funding to inform patients and residents about their treatment decision-making rights. Basically, residents and patients have the right to know about advance directives, their illness (e.g., diagnosis and prognosis), and their treatment options. Patients and residents then have the right to either accept or refuse treatment.

The purpose of the Patient Self Determination Act is to place the treatment decision-making power in the hands of the patient or resident.

Discussion Tips

The questions in this section were not designed to assess CNAs' knowledge concerning the legal issues of patient autonomy. Rather, the objective was to find out how CNAs *feel* about a resident's choice to end aggressive treatment. Therefore, there are no right or wrong answers to these questions. During the educational sessions, however, information about the residents' legal rights to make treatment choices should be emphasized.

We have found in our own work that nurses and CNAs often have ambiguous feelings about the decision to end aggressive medical treatment, in particular feeding tubes. While theoretically CNAs usually recognize the resident's right to make decisions, it is often difficult for them to accept it when the situation actually arises. Discussing difficult cases within the context of patient autonomy may help staff better tolerate decisions they do not agree with. Additionally, when the emphasis of treatment planning is focused on carrying out the wishes of the resident, and the staff is informed and aware that these are the residents' wishes, they are usually more accepting of the decision to withdraw life-sustaining treatment. On the other hand, if staff, in particular CNAs who work so closely with residents, believe a decision not to treat is someone else's (even families'), they feel distressed. Thus, it is important to emphasize that the goal of treatment planning is to protect and carry out the resident's wishes.

To facilitate discussion ask the CNAs whether they had cases in which a resident (or family member) refused life-sustaining treatment. Give the CNAs a few examples of what you mean:

- If a resident needed a feeding tube to stay alive but the family refused to have the feeding tube inserted.
- If the resident had gangrene but refused to have an amputation.
- If the resident refused to continue dialysis.
- If a resident or family member refused all medication other than for the control of pain.

If the CNAs have had these types of cases, ask them to describe the cases and what the outcomes were (did the resident die, did the resident decide to have the treatment in the end?). Ask the CNAs what they thought about the case, what it was like for them to take care of the residents. Did they feel the residents had a comfortable death or an uncomfortable death? Did they feel the residents' wishes were carried out? If so or if not, how did they feel about that?

Discuss with the CNAs that there will be times when residents or their health care agents make decisions that we would not have made or would not have chosen for ourselves but they have the legal right to make those choices. It may be helpful to point out that though we may not understand the decisions that are sometimes made we may appreciate the underlying motivation for those decisions, such as religious beliefs, personal values, comfort, etc.

As discussed previously, protecting the resident's right to make treatment choices will sometimes be difficult for staff. We have to be sensitive to this and provide both formal and informal support on an ongoing basis.

Some of the questions in this section are somewhat repetitive, therefore you may want to just go over a few of them and then come back to the section again during the next session.

QUESTIONS 40 AND 41

Study Findings

CNAs' responses to these questions (Q40 & Q41) indicated that they feel residents should not be forced to continue a treatment they do not want. Seventy-nine percent of CNAs "agreed" that residents should not be forced to take antibiotics and 83% "agreed" residents should not be forced to have a feeding tube. However, when CNAs talked about their own experiences with residents who refused treatment their feelings were dramatically varied.

Case Examples

- One CNA described a very difficult case she was going through at the time of the study: A resident she was taking care of was a 40 year-old woman who could no longer swallow. Most of the members of the resident's family wanted her to have a feeding tube. The husband however was against this and asked the nursing home not to insert a feeding tube. The husband's wishes were respected and the tube was not placed. The CNA was upset by this and she cried while discussing the case. She felt the resident was in pain and starving. She did not know whether the husband was the health care agent and she was not aware of whether or not this was what the resident would want. The CNA said she could not understand why the husband would do this to his wife. A second CNA said another factor which made this case difficult was that the husband did not visit that often anymore. He only came to see his wife about once a month. The CNAs were upset that he was making decisions for the resident without seeing how those decisions were affecting her. The staff, on the other hand, were there to care for the resident every day.
- In another facility there was a case that upset many of the CNAs. A woman developed gangrene in her leg and refused to have an amputation. The resident's family was supportive of her treatment wishes. A number of the CNAs, however, were upset by them. The CNAs felt the resident was depressed and for that reason was refusing the amputation. They thought the family should have convinced her to have the procedure. This case was especially difficult for the CNAs because of the patient's illness. The sight and smell of the gangrene made the work particularly unpleasant. Additionally, the resident was in pain whenever the dressings on her leg were changed. Most of the CNAs who took care of this resident said they tried to make her as comfortable as possible; however, one CNA said she did not take extra care when she was working with the resident because she felt the resident brought the pain on herself by refusing to have the amputation.

These cases indicate that while theoretically CNAs often recognize the residents' right to make treatment decisions (as illustrated by responses to the questionnaire and the general discussion surrounding resident autonomy), when a case actually arises acceptance of treatment termination decisions can be very difficult. CNAs often stated that "I just don't understand why the resident would not want treatment" or "why would they do that to their parent."

On the other hand, there are times when staff are in total agreement with a resident's decision. One such case follows:

- One CNA described a resident she had cared for who refused life-sustaining treatment. The resident was an elderly woman who was dying of cancer. The resident refused to have any treatment or medication that would prolong her life. The CNA said she felt the woman "died with dignity."

QUESTIONS 15 AND 16 (42 AND 43) AGAIN EXAMINE CNAs' FEELINGS TOWARDS TERMINATING LIFE-SUSTAINING TREATMENT, AS WELL AS WHETHER THERE ARE DIFFERENCES IN ATTITUDE BETWEEN STOPPING AND NOT STARTING TREATMENT

Prompt Questions

- Do you think there are times that treatment should not be given? If so, when?
- Is there a difference between not starting a feeding tube and stopping a feeding tube? Is there an emotional difference between the two, does it feel differently or not?

Study Findings

The responses to these questions (Q15 & Q16) were similar to each other. About a third of the CNAs (35%) "agreed" that sometimes a treatment such as a feeding tube should *not be started*, 49% "disagreed," and 16% responded "don't know." Similarly, 30% of CNAs "agreed" that sometimes it is right to *stop* a treatment such as a feeding tube, 55% "disagreed," and 15% were not sure how they felt. During discussions CNAs generally said residents should be given a feeding tube unless the resident specified that he/she would not want one.

Most CNAs felt that there is no real difference between not starting a feeding tube and stopping a feeding tube. CNAs said if a resident wants a feeding tube he/she should get it, however, the resident should not be forced to have it. The resident's preferences should take priority and it should not make a difference whether it is a question of not starting a treatment or stopping a treatment. In a couple of nursing homes, however, CNAs did differentiate between not starting and stopping treatment. These CNAs felt that residents should not be given a feeding tube if they don't want it, however, if the feeding tube has been started it should not be permissible to remove it. Another interesting, though not surprising, finding was CNAs' misperception that once a treatment has been started (particularly a feeding tube) it *cannot legally* be stopped.

Educational Information

Many people believe that once a treatment has been started it cannot be stopped. However, even a feeding tube can be discontinued if this is what the resident desires, if it was indicated in a living will, or if the heath care agent states this is what the resident would want.

There has been some controversy concerning the differences between not starting a feeding tube in the first place versus stopping it once it has already been started. Some people feel that it is more acceptable not to start a treatment and let the illness run its natural course than it is to begin a treatment and then remove it. The removal of a treatment may be perceived as actively doing something which will ultimately result in the resident's death. Therefore it may be more emotionally or psychologically difficult than never having treated. However, from a medical and legal standpoint there is considered to be no difference between not starting a treatment in the first place versus stopping it once it has begun.

The belief that a treatment cannot be terminated once it has been started may result in reluctance on the part of health care agents to have a life-sustaining treatment such as a feeding tube started. For example, consider a case in which an elderly resident has a stroke and can no longer swallow. The resident's daughter (the health care agent) knows that her mother would not want to live for years on a feeding tube. The doctor tells the daughter there is a small chance that over the next six to twelve months her mother may improve substantially and regain the ability to eat by mouth. If the daughter believes that once the feeding tube is placed it cannot be removed she is faced with a difficult dilemma. Should she have the feeding tube inserted when there is a significant likelihood that her mother will never recover and will have to spend the remainder of her life (perhaps years) on a feeding tube which she knows her mother would never want? Or, should she instruct the doctor not to insert the feeding tube thereby eliminating her mother's only chance of survival? Some feel the risk of living for years on a feeding tube is too great and are reluctant to opt for treatment. The option of *time limited trials* (discussed below) presents patients and health care agents with alternative options.

Time Limited Trials

Time limited trials allow the patient the opportunity to recover while maintaining the right to cease treatment if improvement does not occur. With time limited trials the health care team and health care agent agree upon a specified period of time (e.g., two weeks or twelve months, after which recovery would be unlikely) over which the resident will receive the treatment. If the resident improves the treatment is discontinued because it is no longer needed. If after the specified period of time the resident does not improve the resident's condition is reassessed and the treatment can be stopped in the interest of fulfilling the resident's wishes. Thus, with time limited trials the health care agent can feel that the possibility of recovery was not abandoned while at the same time respecting the resident's wishes not to continue a treatment that he/she would not want for a prolonged period of time. Again the resident's religious and cultural values must be taken into account when considering this option. Not all religions find this option permissible particularly when a feeding tube is the treatment under consideration.

QUESTIONS 24 AND 27 EXAMINE WHETHER CNAS FEEL THAT STOPPING LIFE-SUSTAINING TREATMENT IS EQUIVALENT TO KILLING OR ASSISTING THE RESIDENT TO COMMIT SUICIDE

Study Findings

Thirty-three percent of CNAs "agreed" that discontinuing a feeding tube was the same as killing a resident and 53% "agreed" that stopping treatment is the same as assisting suicide.

CNAs who disagreed with these questions generally felt that it was the underlying disease that killed the resident rather than the lack of treatment.

Discussion Tips

Acknowledge that these are difficult questions to answer and that like almost all of the other questions in the questionnaire there are no right or wrong answers. The purpose is to find out how CNAs feel about these issues.

Educational Information

Stopping or not starting a treatment such as a feeding tube in accord with residents' wishes is legally acceptable. Moreover, it is illegal for a facility not to stop or to start a treatment that a resident does not want. On the other hand, physician-assisted suicide is not legal in any state other than Oregon at this time.

QUESTION 22 IS A SUMMARY QUESTION ON THE TOPIC OF PATIENT AUTONOMY

Educational Information

Basically, residents and patients do have the right to refuse life-sustaining treatment, even if refusing such treatment results in death.

Study Findings

Almost all of the CNAs (88%) who took part in the project agreed with this statement, while 6% disagreed and 6% were not sure how they felt about it. Again it should be pointed out that while theoretically CNAs believe in patient autonomy they find it much more difficult to accept when a case actually arises.

Practical Implications for the Nursing Home

Though staff often has difficulty accepting the termination of life-sustaining treatment, this decision is often easier to accept when it is clear that it is the residents' wishes being carried out. A number of CNAs stated that "if it is what the resident wants I am OK with that." Unfortunately, CNAs are usually left out of treatment planning meetings and are not adequately informed concerning why decisions are made. Often CNAs are simply told treatment has been stopped because that is what the family wants. They are not informed whether or not the family member is the health care agent (in which case chosen and trusted by the resident to make health care decisions), whether the resident clearly made the request, and/or any underlying reasons for the request. Thus, CNAs are left to speculate on their own why a family member chose to terminate treatment, sometimes coming to less than favorable conclusions about the relative's motives.

As stated previously CNAs should be included in care planning. In addition to the important information they can provide about residents' conditions, CNAs should be as informed as the rest of the staff concerning the reasons for following a specific treatment pathway. CNAs should feel confident in the knowledge that it is the residents' wishes that are being carried out. In particular, because they are the ones providing the hands-on care during the dying process.

TRUTH-TELLING

Question 21

Prompt Questions

- What is a DNR order?
- Do you think we should talk to residents about things like DNRs, living wills, and health care proxies? Do you think residents should know about their treatment choices?
- Do you think it's better to talk to families instead of the residents themselves about things like living wills, health care proxies, and Do Not Resuscitate orders (DNRs)?
- What do you think is the best way to talk to a resident about a DNR order?

Study Findings

(As compared to their knowledge about health care proxies and living wills, CNAs were much more familiar with DNR orders). CNAs were about equally split on whether or not they thought residents would feel hopeless if they were asked about a DNR. CNAs who thought residents would feel hopeless (42%) generally said discussions about DNRs would depress residents and these types of issues should be discussed with families instead. They said that in general when residents come into nursing homes they feel hopeless and think the nursing home is the last stop before death.

CNAs who disagreed with this statement (39%) said it depends on the resident and how you tell the resident about a DNR. These CNAs said some residents will feel hopeless but others will not. Additionally, they said there is an appropriate way to discuss these types of issues with residents. They felt residents should be educated about advance directives so they can make informed decisions for themselves.

Discussion Tips

Ask CNAs what they think is the appropriate way to discuss DNRs and other advance directives with residents. Let the CNAs know how residents are informed about advance directives in your facility and who is responsible for discussing these issues with the residents. The purpose of this discussion is again to emphasize the issue of resident autonomy. Despite the fact that many of the issues surrounding illness, treatment, and advance directives are difficult to discuss it is important to recognize that residents have the right to know about these topics and make decisions. On the other hand it is important to recognize that while residents have the right to make these decisions they also have the right to postpone decision-making or defer it to someone else.

QUESTION 23

Prompt Questions

- What types of decisions do residents like to leave up to other people?
- Who do residents ask to make decisions for them?
- In the nursing home, what are the things that residents can still decide for themselves?
- In the nursing home, what are the things that residents can no longer make decisions about for themselves?

Study Findings

About half the CNAs (52%) "agreed" that "many residents prefer to let others make decisions for them." They said residents often turn to family members for decisions about treatment. CNAs also said residents will ask them to help make decisions about a wide range of things and sometimes will ask CNAs for their opinions before asking their own families. Usually residents ask CNAs about everyday type matters (e.g., what to wear or what to eat) but sometimes they will request advice on treatment decisions.

CNAs said that while some residents do ask other people to make decisions for them, others have very clear ideas about what they want and make decisions on their own. As a CNA described one resident: "She would tell me to choose whatever dress I thought was best for her to wear—but then when I would choose a dress she would say, 'Oh no! Not that one; choose another,' and I would keep taking dresses out of her closet until I got to the one she wanted. She knew what she wanted to wear."

Discussion Tips

This question (Q23) raises the issue of personal control which residents typically lose to a large extent when entering a nursing home. Discuss the things that residents have to give up and can no longer do. Ask the CNAs what they think it is like for residents when they come into the nursing homes. What are the types of things residents can still make decisions about? Are there ways to give the residents more control over themselves and the environment? Ask about barriers to resident decision-making. As one of the CNAs in our sessions pointed out: "You try to accommodate them as much as possible but you also have take their roommates into account."

QUESTION 29

Prompt Questions

- Do you think most people prefer not to know they are dying?
- Would you want to know if you were dying?
- If you would not want to know you were dying, why wouldn't you want to know?
- If you would want to know you were dying, why would you want to know?

Discussion Tips

The prompt question "would you want to know if you were dying" provides an excellent opportunity to discuss individual differences. Participants are usually very interested in this question and very forthcoming in their point of view. Most will probably state that they would not want to know, but some will most likely say "you know what, I would want to know." After the CNAs talk about the reasons for their feelings raise the point that people have a wide range of feelings towards these types of issues. Some people will want to know everything about their illness and prognosis (and as discussed below have a right to know everything), others might want enough information to obtain treatment but not want any details, and others might not want to know anything about their illness and defer treatment decisions to family members.

Study Findings

Almost three quarters (73%) of the CNAs believed that "residents would prefer not to know they are dying." Some said that even if other people would want to know they are dying, there is no useful purpose in telling elderly residents they are dying. They have already taken care of many of their responsibilities when they came into the nursing home. Other CNAs said that dying residents can often sense it: "they know when they are dying even without anyone telling them."

When asked about their own feelings on the issue, the majority of CNAs reported that, for themselves, they would not want to know if they were dying. Many said "If I knew I was dying I would go sooner" or "I would just worry and be anxious." In contrast, a few CNAs said they would want to know if they were dying. Some of these CNAs said "even though I know I would be scared and upset, especially in the beginning, I would still want to know." CNAs who would want to know typically said they would want to put things in order. This included planning for their children and families, arranging their finances, and making their religious and spiritual peace. Others said they have always worked and they would want to take the opportunity to "live it up in the end."

Educational Information

Residents/patients have a right to know about their treatment options, health, and prognosis. Thus, if a resident wants to know he/she is dying the resident has that right. On the other hand it is important to remember that not everybody desires to have the same amount of information. There is a great deal of variability in the amount of information patients want to know when they have a serious illness or are dying. Ideally, the health care team should try to determine how much information the individual wants and provide it (Buckman, 1992).

Cultural differences often play a factor when these types of decisions are made. In many countries and cultures, the family, rather than the individual, is informed of any terminal diagnosis. These cultural differences should be respected and there should not be an automatic assumption that patient autonomy is equated with full disclosure. Patient autonomy refers to respecting the decisions and preferences of the patient (Pellegrino, 1992).

Similarly, it should not be assumed that individuals with a specific cultural background do not want to be informed of their condition. Each case should be examined individually.

QUESTION 44 EXAMINES WHETHER WE SHOULD GO ALONG WITH FAMILIES' REQUESTS NOT TO TELL RESIDENTS THEY ARE DYING

Prompt Questions

- Let's say a resident asks if she's dying—should we tell her?
- Why do you think a family member might tell us not to tell a resident that he or she is dying? What do you think about that?

Study Findings

The majority of CNAs (70%) felt that we should go along with families and not tell a resident who can understand that he/she is dying. These CNAs felt that "we have to do what the family asks." Many also believed that families know the resident best and know whether the resident can handle the information. About 17% of CNAs "disagreed" with the question and felt residents should be told about their condition. During discussions they basically stated "residents have a right to know what's the matter with them."

Discussion Tips

During the discussion sessions in the original study, CNAs often said it is not their responsibility to tell residents about their condition. Let the CNAs know that this question is not asking whether they themselves are responsible for revealing this information, rather it is asking about whether they feel as a whole the facility (and whoever has the authority within the facility to tell the resident—doctor, nurse, or social worker) has a responsibility to tell the resident about his/her condition.

The following case is an interesting variation on question 47. It examines whether a cognitively intact resident should be informed about the death of a family member.

Case Example

A cognitively intact resident, Mrs. Randal, had a daughter (Sophie) who visited her mother regularly. Sophie had a close relationship with her mother and the staff was very fond of her. When Sophie was diagnosed with cancer she and the rest of her family decided to keep this information from Mrs. Randal. After Sophie passed away the rest of her family believed Mrs. Randal should not be told about Sophie's death. They said "she won't be able to handle it, she will die if we tell her." Whenever Mrs. Randal would ask why Sophie didn't visit, her family told her that Sophie was away on business. To ensure that Mrs. Randal would not overhear the staff discussing Sophie's death they took away Mrs. Randal's hearing aids.

- Before continuing with the case ask the CNAs what they think. Do they think Mrs. Randal should be told about Sophie? What do they think about the removal of the hearing aids? How do they think the situation should be handled?

Case continued: The staff at the nursing home, in particular the CNAs, were upset by the case. They didn't like to lie to Mrs. Randal and they thought she should be able to have her hearing aids. After some discussion the staff decided Mrs. Randal had a right to know about what happened to her daughter. A couple of weeks after Sophie died (the staff wanted to give the family a chance to get over the initial grief) a meeting was held with the family to let them know that the staff felt Mrs. Randal should be told about Sophie. If the family felt they needed help in telling Mrs. Randal members of the staff were prepared to go with them and help break the news. The family, along with a psychiatrist and a nurse, told Mrs. Randal about Sophie. The psychiatrist said Mrs. Randal was very sad but had a normal reaction to the news. In the end the family said they were glad they told Mrs. Randal the truth.

- Again ask the CNAs what they think. Do they think the situation was handled well? It should be acknowledged that every case is different and what worked in one situation will not necessarily be the optimal solution in another situation.

Educational Information

A resident has the right to know about his or her medical condition and treatment. If the resident is cognitively intact the health care staff should discuss options with the resident, not the family or health care agent (although the resident may want to include his or her family in the decision-making process). Moreover, the resident has the right to tell the staff not to discuss his or her condition with the family.

BARRIERS TO CARE

The purpose of this section is to determine the factors that CNAs believe are barriers to the delivery of the best possible patient care.

QUESTION 14 LISTS EIGHT ITEMS THAT ARE POSSIBLE BARRIERS TO CARE

CNAs are asked to indicate how much of a barrier they feel each item is in the delivery of care.

Discussion Tips

Ask the CNAs to discuss which of the items they feel are a problem. Ask whether there are any other things they can think of that prevent residents from getting the best possible care. Ask what might interfere with CNAs being able to provide the best possible care. Is there anything that they think could help them give residents better care?

Study Findings

The following is the percentage of CNAs in the original study that rated each of the items as "very much" a barrier to care:

Percentage of CNAs that rated barrier as "Very Much" a problem

1) Not enough staff   39%
2) Fear of being sued   32%
3) Communication problems among staff   27%
4) Not including all staff in decisions about treatment   25%
5) Communication problems with residents or their families[2]   21%
6) Cost of a treatment   18%
7) Differences of opinion among staff   16%

Not surprisingly, "not enough staff" was rated by the greatest number of CNAs as "very much" a barrier to providing residents with the best possible care. Participants who had been CNAs for many years often stated the work load has increased over the years. They generally have a larger case load of residents than they used to and a greater percentage of residents need total care. Added strain occurs when workers call in sick and other CNAs have to cover their cases. CNAs often said the large workload prevents them from being able to provide residents with as much hands-on care as they would like.

About a third of CNAs said "fear of being sued" is "very much" a barrier to care. There is a prevailing belief that a worker or the facility as a whole can be sued relatively easily. Thus, staff express the feeling that you have to do whatever the family wants even if you do not believe it is in the best interest of the resident. Moreover, it may make CNAs more apprehensive when working in the presence of families.

The next two variables most often rated as "very much" barriers to care were "communication problems among staff" and "not including all staff in decisions about treatment." When discussing both of these items CNAs typically said CNAs are left out of the discussion about treatment. They generally felt that they have valuable information to contribute about the residents. As one CNA stated, "Look, I don't expect or want them to ask me what medication the resident needs, but I can tell them how well the resident can eat, whether she is comfortable, and what she is able to do on her own." In addition to not being asked to contribute information, CNAs often felt they did not receive enough information. They often want to know more about a resident's condition and why different treatments are needed.

One of the main problems talked about in terms of communication was the relaying of information across shifts. CNAs often said that adequate information did not pass from one shift to the other. Additionally, even if the nurses relayed information to each other it often did not get passed on to the CNAs.

About a fifth of CNAs said "communication problems with residents or their families" are "very much" a barrier to care. One of the problems that CNAs identified in this area was abusive treatment by residents and families. CNAs typically reported this to be more of an issue with families than with residents. "If a resident calls you a bad name or says something nasty to you, it's OK. They are sick and they can't help it. It's also really hard for them here and they have no one else to take it out on. But when the families treat you badly—they don't have any excuses."

---

[2]This item has been split into two separate items: one examining communication with residents, the other examining communication with residents' families.

Another difficulty with residents and their families is that they sometimes do not appreciate all of the competing demands on the CNAs. "Families and residents don't want to accept that you have eight or nine other residents that you also need to take care of."

"Cost of a treatment" and "differences of opinion among staff" were not perceived as being as such serious barriers to care as the other items.

FINANCIAL CONCERNS

QUESTION 25 EXAMINES RESIDENTS AND FAMILIES LEGAL RIGHTS CONCERNING OVERTREATMENT

Prompt Questions

- Do you think residents should be allowed to sue doctors or facilities for overtreating?

Study Findings

Fifty-nine percent of CNAs in the original study "agreed" that doctors have been sued by residents and their families for overtreating while 14% "disagreed" and 27% answered "don't know."

Educational Information

Doctors can and have been sued for overtreating. Therefore, nowadays hospitals and nursing homes have to make sure that not only do they give appropriate and adequate treatment, they also have to be careful not to give treatment the patient does not want, even if that treatment is needed to keep the patient alive. Giving a treatment the resident does not want constitutes the crime of battery.

Discussion Tips

Tell the CNAs that this is one of the only questions in the questionnaire that does have a right or wrong answer. Ask CNAs what they think about this. Do they think a resident (or the family) should be able to sue the doctor for trying to keep the resident alive? Discuss that the reason behind these laws is to protect the resident's rights. Even if the doctor feels he/she knows what's right for the resident it is legally the right of the resident (or those closest to the resident) to make these types of decisions.

QUESTION 32 EXAMINES CNAS' ATTITUDES TOWARDS PROVIDING THE ELDERLY WITH EXPENSIVE MEDICAL TREATMENT

Study Findings

Most CNAs (81%) "disagreed" that we should *not* use very expensive treatment to keep very old people alive, while only 8% agreed and 11% responded "don't know." CNAs typically said everyone is entitled to treatment and people should not be discriminated against because of their age.

CNAs were also asked what they think should happen if there are situations of limited resources. For example, should older people receive costly treatments such as transplants when only a small number of them can be done? Although a few CNAs said they feel young children should receive treatment before the elderly, most CNAs stated that they felt as long as the older person can tolerate treatment he/she is entitled to it. They felt allocation of resources should be determined on a first come, first serve basis.

THE CNA AS PART OF THE HEALTH CARE TEAM

QUESTIONS 34, 45, 46, AND 47

Prompt Questions

- Do you feel other CNAs value your opinions?
- Other than your fellow CNAs, do you feel the people you work with value your opinion?

Study Findings

Question 34—A little less than half (46%) of the CNAs "agreed" that their opinions are valued by those they work with, while 34% "disagreed" and 20% said they "don't know." During the discussion sessions, most though not all CNAs said their opinions are respected by the other CNAs. There was less agreement concerning whether other staff (in particular the discussion focused on nurses) valued CNAs' opinions. Some CNAs were confident that nurses listened to what they had to say about residents, while others felt they were looked down upon by the nursing staff (this is discussed in more detail below).

Discussion Tips

Questions 45, 46, and 47 allow for a more in-depth examination of how the CNAs feel about their interactions with different members of the health care team as well as residents and their families.

In the original study Questions 45, 46, and 47 were combined into one question. The original question asked how satisfied CNAs were with their opportunities to discuss residents' treatment with different members of the health care team, residents, and families. We felt it was important to look at this issue in more detail. Questions 45, 46, and 47 are designed to help determine where and why breakdown in communication may occur.

Study Findings

During discussion CNAs typically stated they felt that they are at the bottom of the nursing home hierarchy and are left out of discussions about resident care and treatment.

(Q45A) Doctors—Most CNAs said doctors never ask them about treatment and many said the only time the doctor talks to them is to ask where is the resident's chart. "The doctors don't see us." "They don't realize they get their information from us. Nurses ask us about the residents and the doctors ask the nurses."

(Q45B) Nurses—From among all the staff CNAs were most satisfied with their discussions with nurses. Many CNAs said nurses ask them about residents and listen to their input. They felt the nurses on their floors were good to work with and cared about the residents. Others, however, felt that nurses only listen and ask questions when there is a problem. They said the early warning signs they relayed to nurses about residents were generally ignored. One CNA said a nurse told her, "I didn't go to nursing school to listen to a CNA."

(Q45C) Social Workers—Surprisingly, at most facilities CNAs said they had little contact with social workers. Occasionally, social workers provided support when residents died, however, it was rare for CNAs to say that a social worker asked them for information about the residents. CNAs felt they could provide valuable information to social workers, particularly concerning the social behaviors of residents. For example, CNAs often said they can tell which residents would make good roommates but the social workers never ask for their advice.

(Q45D) Clergy—A large percentage of CNAs were not satisfied with their interactions with clergy but this was largely due to lack of opportunity. CNAs typically did not have much contact with clergy.

(Q45E) Administrators—Forty percent of CNAs reported not being satisfied with their interactions with administrators. A common grievance was that administration does not protect the CNAs from resident and family complaints. "The administration always believes the resident, even when the resident is confused. Why don't we have any rights?" It should be pointed out however, that at a few facilities, CNAs did feel supported by administration, particularly nursing administration, and were thankful for the support.

(Q45F) Residents—Many CNAS have close relationships with their residents. CNAs who were not satisfied with interactions with residents often said residents do not appreciate the fact that CNAs have at least eight other residents for whom they are responsible.

(Q45G) Families—CNAs said they are not allowed to talk to families about any aspect of the residents' medical condition. While CNAs felt they should be allowed more freedom when talking to families, most stated they would not want the responsibility of talking to families about the more complex aspects of residents' condition and treatment.

The quality of CNAs' reported interactions with families varied greatly. The following are some examples of these interactions:

- "Some families are very nice and appreciative and make you feel good about your job."
- "When a resident dies you also lose the family and that can be really hard too. You get close to families."
- "Families sometimes talk to us like we are the maids who don't know anything."

CNAS' DEGREE OF COMFORT WITH CARING FOR RESIDENTS WHO ARE NOT RECEIVING TREATMENT

QUESTIONS 35 AND 36

Prompt Question

- Does it make a difference whether the resident or the health care agent (e.g., daughter, spouse, or nephew) made the choice to stop treatment?

Study Findings

Seventeen percent of CNAs "agreed" that they are "not comfortable caring for residents who will die because they are refusing life-sustaining treatment." Slightly more (21%) "agreed" that they are "not comfortable caring for a resident who will die because their health care agents are refusing life-sustaining treatment." CNAs generally said that they will continue to care for residents and make them as comfortable as possible even when they are refusing treatment.

Discussion

These questions were designed to examine two issues: 1) Are CNAS comfortable caring for residents who are not receiving life-sustaining treatment, and 2) Does it matter whether it is the resident's or the health care agent's decision not to continue life-sustaining treatment. In the original study slightly more CNAs "agreed" that they were uncomfortable when the health care agent made the decision than when the resident made the decision. Discuss this issue with the CNAs and ask them whether they feel it matters whether it is the agent or the resident. Reinforce to the CNAs that the person who is the health care agent was personally chosen by the resident to make health care decisions, and is therefore trusted by the resident.

SUMMARY

The following is a summary of the important points covered during the educational/discussion sessions. Give each of the CNAs a copy of the summary and go over each point together with the CNAs. This should only take about 5 to 10 minutes.

SUMMARY

1. Autonomy of the resident

   - Patient Self Determination Act (1991)—residents have the right to accept or refuse treatment.
   - Recognition that choices made by residents may be difficult for family and/or staff. Family and staff should be supported through these difficult times.

2. Advance Directives

   - Health Care Proxy/Durable Power of Attorney for Health Care
   - Living Will

3. Truth-Telling

   - Residents have the right to know about their condition.

- The amount of information a person wants to know about their own condition will depend on the person. The health care staff should try to determine the amount of information the person wants to know and provide that information.

4. Comfort Care

- It is possible to keep most dying patients from feeling much pain.
- Often patients do not get adequate pain relief:

—fear of patient becoming addicted
—fear of hastening death of patient
—not paying enough attention to signs which would indicate the patient is in pain (especially among dementia patients).

- Stopping aggressive medical treatment does not mean an end to all treatment or to care. Residents are especially in need of comfort care at this time!
- Comfort care needs:

Positioning
Hygiene needs
Dressings
Cold compresses
Mouth care
Touch
Talking to residents

7
Posttest Session (Optional)

A posttest session can be used to determine changes in knowledge and attitude. This can be done by re-administering the Ethics Questionnaire in Appendix A. Additionally, following the administration of the questionnaires ask the CNAs what they thought about this program, did they feel it was helpful, are there other issues that they would have liked to discuss. The Ethics Education Evaluation Form can also be used to obtain CNAs' evaluation of the program (found in Appendix D).

APPENDIXES

APPENDICES

Appendix A
Ethics Questionnaire

R# _ _ _ _ _

Some nursing home residents have health care proxies and/or living wills in case a time ever comes when they can no longer make decisions on their own. Please circle "yes," "no," or "don't know" to the questions about health care proxies and living wills. If you are not sure about a certain question or don't know what a "health care proxy" or "living will" is, either circle "don't know" or give it your best guess. Don't worry if you don't know the answers to these questions. Many people do not know about health care proxies and living wills. We will spend time discussing living wills and health care proxies during the first discussion session.

1. Can the health care agent (the person named in the health care proxy form) make financial decisions for the resident?
   - 1 YES
   - 2 NO
   - 3 DON'T KNOW

2. Can the health care agent tell the doctor not to give the resident antibiotics when the resident has pneumonia?
   - 1 YES
   - 2 NO
   - 3 DON'T KNOW

3. Can the health care agent sell the resident's home or apartment?
   - 1 YES
   - 2 NO
   - 3 DON'T KNOW

4. Can the health care agent ask the doctor *to stop* a tube feeding once it has already begun?
   - 1 YES
   - 2 NO
   - 3 DON'T KNOW

5. Can a health care agent ask the doctor *not to start* a tube feeding if the resident can no longer eat by mouth?

    1 YES
    2 NO
    3 DON'T KNOW

6. Can a health care agent sign permission for an amputation if the resident has gangrene?

    1 YES
    2 NO
    3 DON'T KNOW

7. If a resident left instructions (for example made out a living will) that he would not want to be fed by feeding tube if he could no longer swallow food and would never regain the ability to swallow food—could the nursing home give him a feeding tube anyway?

    1 YES
    2 NO
    3 DON'T KNOW

8. If a resident left instructions (made out a living will) that she would not want to have any amputations—could a doctor perform an amputation if the resident gets gangrene?

    1 YES
    2 NO
    3 DON'T KNOW

*9. If there is no living will and no health care proxy can the family make the decision to stop a feeding tube?

    1 YES
    2 NO
    3 DON'T KNOW

*10. If there is no living will and no health care proxy can the doctor make a decision to stop a feeding tube?

    1 YES
    2 NO
    3 DON'T KNOW

11. What is a health care proxy? _____
_____

12. What is a living will? _____
_____

Question 13 examines resident, family, and staff support.

13a. At this nursing home, do you think the staff tries to find out what kinds of treatment very sick residents want?

---

*The answers to questions 9 and 10 are state dependent. You may wish to skip these questions.

1 ALWAYS OR ALMOST ALWAYS
2 SOMETIMES
3 NEVER OR ALMOST NEVER
4 DON'T KNOW

13b. At this nursing home, do you think that when residents become ill, they or the person responsible for them are told about the different choices they have as far as different types of treatments are concerned?

1 ALWAYS OR ALMOST ALWAYS
2 SOMETIMES
3 NEVER OR ALMOST NEVER
4 DON'T KNOW

13c. At this nursing home, do you think that when residents become ill, they or the person responsible for them are helped to make a decision about treatment?

1 ALWAYS OR ALMOST ALWAYS
2 SOMETIMES
3 NEVER OR ALMOST NEVER
4 DON'T KNOW

13d. At this nursing home, do you think families of residents who are dying get emotional support or counseling?

1 ALWAYS OR ALMOST ALWAYS
2 SOMETIMES
3 NEVER OR ALMOST NEVER
4 DON'T KNOW

13e. At this nursing home, do you feel that when you are caring for a resident who is dying, you (the staff) get some kind of emotional support or counseling?

1 ALWAYS OR ALMOST ALWAYS
2 SOMETIMES
3 NEVER OR ALMOST NEVER
4 DON'T KNOW

14. How much do you think each of the following things prevents residents in this nursing home from getting the best possible care? (Circle the number that best describes what you think.)

	NOT AT ALL	SOME-WHAT	VERY MUCH
a. Differences of opinion among staff.	1	2	3
b. Not including all staff in the decisions about treatment.	1	2	3
c. Fear of being sued.	1	2	3
d. How much something will cost.	1	2	3
e. Not enough staff.	1	2	3

		NOT AT ALL	SOME-WHAT	VERY MUCH
f.	Communication problems among the staff.	1	2	3
g.	Communication problems with residents.	1	2	3
h.	Communication problems with residents' families.	1	2	3

Many of the following statements have no wrong or right answers, but are simply trying to find out how most people feel about certain issues. For each of the statements, circle the answer that best describes how *you* feel.

15. Sometimes there are acceptable reasons *not to start* a treatment, such as a feeding tube, even if it means a resident may die sooner.
> 1 AGREE
> 2 DISAGREE
> 3 DON'T KNOW

16. Sometimes there are acceptable reasons to *stop* a treatment, such as a feeding tube, even if it means a resident may die sooner.
> 1 AGREE
> 2 DISAGREE
> 3 DON'T KNOW

17a. A dying person should always be offered food.
> 1 AGREE
> 2 DISAGREE
> 3 DON'T KNOW

17b. A dying person should always be offered water.
> 1 AGREE
> 2 DISAGREE
> 3 DON'T KNOW

18. A dying person should always receive food and water, even by feeding tube if necessary.
> 1 AGREE
> 2 DISAGREE
> 3 DON'T KNOW

19. Sometimes we make dying residents uncomfortable by continuing to give them food and water by mouth.
> 1 AGREE
> 2 DISAGREE
> 3 DON'T KNOW

20a. Sometimes we make dying residents uncomfortable by giving them tube feedings.

        1 AGREE
        2 DISAGREE
        3 DON'T KNOW

20b. Sometimes we make dying residents uncomfortable by giving them IVs.

        1 AGREE
        2 DISAGREE
        3 DON'T KNOW

21. If you talk to residents about a DNR (Do Not Resuscitate) order they will think their condition is hopeless.

        1 AGREE
        2 DISAGREE
        3 DON'T KNOW

22. All residents who are able to make decisions for themselves have the right to refuse life-saving treatment, even if refusing such treatment may result in death.

        1 AGREE
        2 DISAGREE
        3 DON'T KNOW

23. Residents usually prefer to let other people make decisions for them.

        1 AGREE
        2 DISAGREE
        3 DON'T KNOW

24. Letting patients die by not giving them a certain treatment is the same thing as helping them to commit suicide.

        1 AGREE
        2 DISAGREE
        3 DON'T KNOW

25. Some residents or their families have sued doctors when the residents were given a treatment to keep them alive that they did not want.

        1 AGREE
        2 DISAGREE
        3 DON'T KNOW

26. It is possible to prevent dying residents from feeling much pain.

        1 AGREE
        2 DISAGREE
        3 DON'T KNOW

27. Stopping a feeding tube is the same as killing a resident.

        1 AGREE
        2 DISAGREE
        3 DON'T KNOW

28. Sometimes it is right to give pain medication to relieve suffering, even if it may make a person die sooner.
>1 AGREE
>2 DISAGREE
>3 DON'T KNOW

29. Most patients prefer not to know they are dying.
>1 AGREE
>2 DISAGREE
>3 DON'T KNOW

30. If a resident is not able to make decisions (for example, if the resident has Alzheimer's disease), the *doctor* is the best person to make treatment decisions for the resident.
>1 AGREE
>2 DISAGREE
>3 DON'T KNOW

31. If a resident is not able to make decision (for example, if the resident has Alzheimer's disease), a *family member* is the best person to make decisions for the resident.
>1 AGREE
>2 DISAGREE
>3 DON'T KNOW

32. We should not use expensive treatments to keep very old people alive.
>1 AGREE
>2 DISAGREE
>3 DON'T KNOW

33. In this nursing home, the spiritual needs of dying residents receive too little attention.
>1 AGREE
>2 DISAGREE
>3 DON'T KNOW

34. My opinions about what should be done for residents are valued by the people I work with.
>1 AGREE
>2 DISAGREE
>3 DON'T KNOW

35. I am not comfortable caring for residents who will most likely die because *they* are refusing life-sustaining treatment.
>1 AGREE
>2 DISAGREE
>3 DON'T KNOW

36. I am not comfortable caring for residents who will most likely die because *their health care agents* (the people responsible for the residents, for example, the family members) are refusing life-sustaining treatment.

1 AGREE
2 DISAGREE
3 DON'T KNOW

37. Sometimes I feel the treatments we give the residents are too uncomfortable for them.
   1 AGREE
   2 DISAGREE
   3 DON'T KNOW

38. If a resident wants antibiotics in order to be kept alive the nursing home should provide the antibiotics.
   1 AGREE
   2 DISAGREE
   3 DON'T KNOW

39. If a resident wants a feeding tube in order to be kept alive the nursing home should provide it.
   1 AGREE
   2 DISAGREE
   3 DON'T KNOW

40. If a resident does not want antibiotics and wants to die, the nursing home should not force the resident to have the treatment.
   1 AGREE
   2 DISAGREE
   3 DON'T KNOW

41. If a resident does not want a tube feeding and wants to die, the nursing home should not force the resident to have the treatment.
   1 AGREE
   2 DISAGREE
   3 DON'T KNOW

42. Even if the resident doesn't want antibiotics, it is wrong to stop them if the antibiotics are keeping the resident alive.
   1 AGREE
   2 DISAGREE
   3 DON'T KNOW

43. Even if the resident doesn't want a feeding tube, it is wrong to stop it if the feeding tube is keeping the resident alive.
   1 AGREE
   2 DISAGREE
   3 DON'T KNOW

44. If a family asks us not to tell a resident, *who can understand,* that he or she has an illness and a certain amount of time to live, we should go along with the family's request and not tell the resident.

1 AGREE
2 DISAGREE
3 DON'T KNOW

45. Do the following people ever ask your opinion about how a resident you are caring for is doing?

		Never	Some- times	Often
a.	Doctors	1	2	3
b.	Nurses	1	2	3
c.	Social workers	1	2	3
d.	Clergy	1	2	3
e.	Administrators	1	2	3
f.	The resident	1	2	3
g.	The resident's family	1	2	3

46. If you were worried about a resident's condition, how likely would you be to tell each of the following people about the resident?

		Not at all likely	Some- what likely	Very likely
a.	Doctors	1	2	3
b.	Nurses	1	2	3
c.	Social workers	1	2	3
d.	Clergy	1	2	3
e.	Administrators	1	2	3
f.	The resident	1	2	3
g.	The resident's family	1	2	3

47. If you were worried about a resident's condition, how comfortable would you feel speaking to each of the following about the resident?

		Never	Some- times	Often
a.	Doctors	1	2	3
b.	Nurses	1	2	3
c.	Social workers	1	2	3
d.	Clergy	1	2	3

e.	Administrators	1	2	3
f.	The resident	1	2	3
g.	The resident's family	1	2	3

48. At this nursing home, who do you think most often makes the final treatment decisions for residents who can't make decisions on their own and might need to be fed by feeding tubes and IVS? (You can circle more than one answer if you wish.)

> 1 THE FAMILY
> 2 THE DOCTOR
> 3 SOMEONE ELSE _____
> (If it is someone else please write down who it is.)

49. Who do you think should make the final treatment decision for residents who can't make decisions and need to be fed by feeding tubes and IVS? (You can circle more than one answer if you wish.)

> 1 THE FAMILY
> 2 THE DOCTOR
> 3 SOMEONE ELSE _____
> (If it is someone else please write down who it is.)

50. If the resident can no longer make decisions, do you think the family should be able to make decisions about treatment when there is no health care proxy and no living will (meaning do you think the family should be allowed to make decisions even if the resident didn't leave them specific instructions)?

> 1 YES
> 2 NO

51. Do you agree that when a resident *is able* to make decisions about life-threatening conditions (for example, if they have pneumonia but ask not to be treated with antibiotics), that their family should be allowed to overrule the resident's decision?

> 1 YES
> 2 NO

52. Have you ever taken care of a resident who refused to have medical treatment that was needed to keep him or her alive (or a resident whose family refused treatment)? Examples include, a resident who refused antibiotics, amputation, dialysis, feeding tube, or any other life-saving medication without which he would die, or a family which refused to allow a treatment when the person needed it to stay alive. This does not include situations when residents are taken off feeding tubes because they have regained the ability to swallow.

> 1 YES
> 2 NO
> 3 DON'T KNOW

Appendix B
Blank Ethics Education Instruction Booklet

HEALTH CARE PROXIES[1] AND LIVING WILLS

Can a health care agent (the person named in the health care proxy) make the following decisions:

	YES	NO	DON'T KNOW
Sell Home (3)			
Financial (1)			
Antibiotics (2)			
Amputate (6)			
Stop Feeding Tube (4)			
Not Start Feeding Tube (5)			

If a resident left a living will saying he/she doesn't want a feeding tube or an amputation, can the doctor:

	YES	NO	DON'T KNOW
Amputate (8)			
Give Feeding Tube (7)			

If there is no living will and no health care proxy can:

	YES	NO	DON'T KNOW
the doctor decide to stop a feeding tube? (10)			

---

[1]This is equivalent to a durable power of attorney in most states.

N.B. Numbers in parentheses refer to item numbers in original questionnaire.

the family decide to stop a
feeding tube? (9)

WHO SHOULD MAKE DECISIONS FOR RESIDENTS?

Do you think the family should be able to make treatment decisions if there is no health care proxy (HCP) and no living will? (50)

     YES   NO   MISSING

In this nursing home, who usually makes the final decision for mentally impaired residents who might need to be fed by feeding tube or IV? (48)

Family

Doctor

Doctor and Family

Other

Who do you think should make these decisions? (49)

Family

Doctor

Doctor and Family

Other

If the resident has Alzheimer's Disease, who is the best person to make decisions for the resident?

                                  AGREE   DISAGREE   DON'T KNOW

Doctor (30)

Family (31)

Should families be able to overrule residents who can make decisions concerning life-threatening conditions (for example if they have pneumonia but ask not to be treated with antibiotics)? (51)

     YES   NO   MISSING

SUPPORT FOR RESIDENTS, STAFF, AND FAMILIES

	ALWAYS	SOMETIMES	NEVER	DON'T KNOW
Staff tries to find out the treatment very sick residents want. (13a)				

	ALWAYS	SOMETIMES	NEVER	DON'T KNOW
Residents and their HCPs are told about treatment choices. (13b)				
Residents and their HCPs are helped to make decisions. (13c)				
Families of dying residents get emotional support or counseling. (13d)				
Staff gets emotional support or counseling. (13e)				

COMFORT ISSUES

Sometimes I feel the treatments we give residents are too uncomfortable. (37)

    AGREE   DISAGREE   DON'T KNOW

Sometimes we make dying residents more uncomfortable by continuing to give them food and water by mouth. (19)

    AGREE   DISAGREE   DON'T KNOW

Sometimes we make dying residents more uncomfortable by giving them feeding tubes. (20a)

    AGREE   DISAGREE   DON'T KNOW

Sometimes we make dying residents more uncomfortable by giving them IVs. (20b)

    AGREE   DISAGREE   DON'T KNOW

It is possible to prevent a dying resident from feeling much pain. (26)

    AGREE   DISAGREE   DON'T KNOW

Sometimes it is right to give pain medication even if the person may die sooner. (28)

    AGREE   DISAGREE   DON'T KNOW

In this nursing home, the spiritual needs of dying residents receive too little attention. (33)

    AGREE   DISAGREE   DON'T KNOW

A dying person should always be offered food. (17a)

    AGREE   DISAGREE   DON'T KNOW

A dying person should always be offered water. (17b)

    AGREE   DISAGREE   DON'T KNOW

A dying person should always receive food and water, even by feeding tube if necessary. (18)

    AGREE   DISAGREE   DON'T KNOW

AUTONOMY AND TREATMENT

If a resident wants antibiotics in order to be kept alive, the home should provide them. (38)

    AGREE   DISAGREE   DON'T KNOW

If a resident wants a feeding tube in order to be kept alive, the home should provide it. (39)

    AGREE   DISAGREE   DON'T KNOW

If a resident doesn't want antibiotics and wants to die, the home shouldn't force the resident to have them. (40)

    AGREE   DISAGREE   DON'T KNOW

If a resident doesn't want a feeding tube and wants to die, the nursing home shouldn't force the resident to have it. (41)

    AGREE   DISAGREE   DON'T KNOW

Sometimes there are acceptable reasons *not to start* a treatment, such as a feeding tube, even if it means a resident may die sooner. (15)

    AGREE   DISAGREE   DON'T KNOW

Sometimes there are acceptable reasons to *stop* a treatment, such as a feeding tube, even if it means a resident may die sooner. (16)

    AGREE   DISAGREE   DON'T KNOW

Even if a resident doesn't want antibiotics, it's wrong to stop them if the antibiotics are needed to keep the resident alive. (42)

    AGREE   DISAGREE   DON'T KNOW

Even if a resident doesn't want a feeding tube, it's wrong to stop it if the feeding tube is keeping the resident alive. (43)

    AGREE   DISAGREE   DON'T KNOW

Not giving treatment is the same as assisting suicide. (24)

        AGREE   DISAGREE   DON'T KNOW

Discontinuing a feeding tube is the same as killing a resident. (27)

        AGREE   DISAGREE   DON'T KNOW

All residents who are able to make decisions for themselves have the right to refuse life-saving treatment, even if refusing such treatment may result in death. (22)

        AGREE   DISAGREE   DON'T KNOW

TRUTH-TELLING

If you talk to a resident about a DNR (Do Not Resuscitate) order, they will think their condition is hopeless. (21)

        AGREE   DISAGREE   DON'T KNOW

Residents usually prefer to let others make decisions for them. (23)

        AGREE   DISAGREE   DON'T KNOW

Most patients prefer not to know they are dying. (29)

        AGREE   DISAGREE   DON'T KNOW

If a family asks us not to tell a resident, *who can understand,* that he/she is dying, should we go along with the request? (44)

        AGREE   DISAGREE   DON'T KNOW

SITUATIONS THAT MIGHT PREVENT STAFF FROM MAKING THE BEST POSSIBLE TREATMENT DECISION FOR RESIDENTS

	NOT AT ALL	SOME- WHAT	VERY MUCH	MISSING
Difference of opinion among staff. (14a)				
Not including all staff in decisions about treatment. (14b)				
Cost. (14c)				
Fear of being sued. (14d)				
Not enough staff. (14e)				

	NOT AT ALL	SOME-WHAT	VERY MUCH	MISSING

Communication problems among staff. (14f)

Communication problems with residents. (14g)

Communication problems with residents' families. (14h)

FINANCIAL CONCERNS

Some doctors have been sued by residents or their families for overtreating. (25)

    AGREE   DISAGREE   DON'T KNOW

We should not use very expensive treatments to keep very old people alive. (32)

    AGREE   DISAGREE   DON'T KNOW

THE CNA AS PART OF THE HEALTH CARE TEAM

My opinions about what should be done for residents are valued by the people I work with. (34)

    AGREE   DISAGREE   DON'T KNOW

Do the following people ask your opinion about how a resident you are caring for is doing?

	NEVER	SOMETIMES	OFTEN	MISSING

Doctors (45a)

Nurses (45b)

Social Workers (45c)

Clergy (45d)

Administrators (45e)

Residents (45f)

Resident's Family (45g)

If you were worried about a resident's condition, how likely would you be to tell each of the following people about the resident?

	NEVER	SOMETIMES	OFTEN	MISSING

Doctors (46a)

Nurses (46b)

	NEVER	SOMETIMES	OFTEN	MISSING
Social Workers (46c)				
Clergy (46d)				
Administrators (46e)				
Residents (46f)				
Resident's Family (46g)				

If you were worried about a resident's condition, how comfortable would you feel speaking to each of the following about the resident?

	NEVER	SOMETIMES	OFTEN	MISSING
Doctors (47a)				
Nurses (47b)				
Social Workers (47c)				
Clergy (47d)				
Administrators (47e)				

	NEVER	SOMETIMES	OFTEN	MISSING
Residents (47f)				
Resident's Family (47g)				

PERSONAL CONCERNS

I am not comfortable caring for residents who will die because *they* are refusing life-sustaining treatment. (35)

AGREE   DISAGREE   DON'T KNOW

I am not comfortable caring for residents who will die because *their health care agents* refuse life-sustaining treatment. (36)

AGREE   DISAGREE   DON'T KNOW

Appendix C

Ethics Education Instruction Booklet containing the percent responses of all CNAs who took part in the Original Greenwall Study[1]

HEALTH CARE PROXIES[2] AND LIVING WILLS

Can a health care agent (the person named in the health care proxy) make the following decisions:

	YES	NO	DON'T KNOW
Sell Home (3)	34%	41%	25%
Financial (1)	55%	21%	24%
Antibiotics (2)	55%	24%	21%
Amputate (6)	59%	19%	22%
Stop Feeding Tube (4)	56%	24%	20%
Not Start Feeding Tube (5)	60%	20%	20%

If a resident left a living will saying he/she doesn't want a feeding tube or an amputation, can the doctor:

	YES	NO	DON'T KNOW
Amputate (8)	10%	79%	11%
Give Feeding Tube (7)	9%	83%	9%

---

[1]Some of these questions have been changed for the current form of the Ethics Questionnaire.

[2]This is equivalent to a durable power of attorney in most states.

189

If there is no living will and no health care proxy can:

	YES	NO	DON'T KNOW
the doctor decide to stop a tube feeding? (9)	52%	33%	15%
the family decide to stop a tube feeding? (10)	67%	23%	10%

WHO SHOULD MAKE DECISIONS FOR RESIDENTS?

Do you think the family should be able to make treatment decisions if there is no health care proxy (HCP) and no living will? (50)

YES	NO	MISSING
82%	13%	5%

In this nursing home, who usually makes the final decision for mentally impaired residents who might need to be fed by feeding tube or IV? (48)

Family	39%
Doctor	34%
Both	20%
Other	3%

Who do you think should make these decisions? (49)

Family	42%
Doctor	32%
Both	18%
Other	2%

If the resident has Alzheimer's Disease, who is the best person to make decisions for the resident?

	AGREE	DISAGREE	DON'T KNOW
Doctor (30)	40%	49%	11%
Family (31)	73%	16%	11%

Should families be able to overrule residents who can make decisions concerning life-threatening conditions (for example, if they have pneumonia but ask not to be treated with antibiotics)? (51)

YES	NO	MISSING
30%	65%	6%

SUPPORT FOR RESIDENTS, STAFF, AND FAMILIES

	ALWAYS	SOMETIMES	NEVER	DON'T KNOW
Staff tries find out the treatment very sick residents want. (13a)	51%	29%	6%	14%
Residents and their HCPs are told about treatment choices. (13b)	63%	16%	1%	19%
Residents and their HCPs are helped to make decisions. (13c)	53%	22%	3%	21%
Families of dying residents get emotional support or counseling. (13d)	55%	24%	3%	18%
Staff gets emotional support or counseling. (13e)	18%	26%	42%	14%

COMFORT ISSUES

Sometimes I feel the treatments we give residents are too uncomfortable. (37)

AGREE	DISAGREE	DON'T KNOW
40%	44%	16%

Sometimes we make dying residents more uncomfortable by continuing to give them food and water by mouth. (19)

AGREE	DISAGREE	DON'T KNOW
56%	27%	18%

Sometimes we make dying residents more uncomfortable by giving them feeding tubes and IVs. (20)

AGREE	DISAGREE	DON'T KNOW
42%	38%	20%

It is possible to prevent a dying resident from feeling much pain. (26)

AGREE	DISAGREE	DON'T KNOW
63%	20%	17%

Sometimes it is right to give pain medication even if the person will die sooner. (28)

AGREE	DISAGREE	DON'T KNOW
53%	29%	18%

In this nursing home, the spiritual needs of dying residents receive too little attention. (33)

AGREE	DISAGREE	DON'T KNOW
30%	55%	16%

A dying person should always be offered food and water by mouth. (17)

AGREE	DISAGREE	DON'T KNOW
52%	38%	10%

A dying person should always receive food and water, even by feeding tube if necessary. (18)

AGREE	DISAGREE	DON'T KNOW
62%	29%	10%

AUTONOMY AND TREATMENT

If a resident wants antibiotics in order to be kept alive, the home should provide them. (38)

AGREE	DISAGREE	DON'T KNOW
76%	10%	14%

If a resident wants a feeding tube in order to be kept alive, the home should provide it. (39)

AGREE	DISAGREE	DON'T KNOW
82%	8%	9%

If a resident doesn't want antibiotics and wants to die, the home shouldn't force the resident to have them. (40)

AGREE	DISAGREE	DON'T KNOW
79%	11%	10%

If a resident doesn't want a feeding tube and wants to die, the nursing home shouldn't force the resident to have it. (41)

AGREE	DISAGREE	DON'T KNOW
83%	9%	8%

Sometimes it is right *not to start* a treatment, such as a feeding tube, even if it means a resident may die sooner. (15)

AGREE	DISAGREE	DON'T KNOW
35%	49%	16%

Sometimes it is right to *stop* a treatment, such as a feeding tube, even if it means a resident may die sooner. (16)

AGREE	DISAGREE	DON'T KNOW
30%	55%	15%

It's wrong to stop antibiotics, if they will keep the resident alive even if he/she doesn't want them. (42)

AGREE	DISAGREE	DON'T KNOW
34%	46%	20%

It's wrong to stop a tube feeding, if it will keep the resident alive even if he/she doesn't want it. (43)

AGREE	DISAGREE	DON'T KNOW
37%	44%	19%

Not giving treatment is the same as assisting suicide. (24)

AGREE	DISAGREE	DON'T KNOW
53%	35%	12%

Discontinuing a feeding tube is the same as killing a resident. (27)

AGREE	DISAGREE	DON'T KNOW
33%	53%	13%

All residents who are able to make decisions for themselves have the right to refuse life-saving treatment, even if refusing such treatment may result in death. (22)

AGREE	DISAGREE	DON'T KNOW
89%	6%	5%

TRUTH-TELLING

If you talk to a resident about a DNR (Do Not Resuscitate) order, they will think their condition is hopeless. (21)

AGREE	DISAGREE	DON'T KNOW
42%	39%	19%

Many residents prefer to let others make decisions for them. (23)

AGREE	DISAGREE	DON'T KNOW
52%	33%	15%

Many patients prefer not to know they are dying. (29)

AGREE	DISAGREE	DON'T KNOW
73%	16%	11%

If a family asks us not to tell a resident, *who can understand*, that he/she is dying, should we go along with the request? (44)

AGREE	DISAGREE	DON'T KNOW
70%	17%	12%

SITUATIONS WHICH MIGHT PREVENT STAFF FROM MAKING THE BEST POSSIBLE TREATMENT DECISION FOR RESIDENTS

	NOT AT ALL	SOMEWHAT	VERY MUCH	MISSING
Lack of knowledge about all possible choices. (14b)	29%	39%	15%	17%
Not enough staff. (14f)	20%	25%	39%	16%
Not including all staff in decisions about treatment. (14c)	31%	30%	25%	15%
Difference of opinion among staff. (14a)	28%	45%	16%	11%
Communication problems among staff. (14g)	23%	37%	27%	14%
	NOT AT ALL	SOMEWHAT	VERY MUCH	MISSING
Communication problems with residents or their families. (14h)	27%	39%	21%	13%
Cost. (14e)	32%	28%	18%	22%
Fear of being sued. (14d)	22%	27%	32%	18%

FINANCIAL CONCERNS

Some doctors have been sued by residents or their families for overtreating. (25)

AGREE	DISAGREE	DON'T KNOW
59%	14%	27%

We should not use very expensive treatments to keep very old people alive. (32)

AGREE	DISAGREE	DON'T KNOW
8%	81%	11%

THE CNA AS PART OF THE HEALTH CARE TEAM

My opinions about what should be done for residents are valued by the people I work with. (34)

AGREE	DISAGREE	DON'T KNOW
46%	34%	20%

SATISFACTION WITH DISCUSSING PATIENT TREATMENT WITH OTHER STAFF

	NOT SATISFIED	SOMEWHAT SATISFIED	VERY SATISFIED	MISSING
Doctors (45a)	39%	22%	19%	20%
Nurses (45b)	16%	36%	35%	12%
Social Workers (45c)	30%	29%	22%	19%
Clergy (45d)	41%	18%	13%	18%
Administrators (45e)	40%	22%	14%	25%
	NOT SATISFIED	SOMEWHAT SATISFIED	VERY SATISFIED	MISSING
Residents (45f)	29%	27%	24%	20%
Resident's Family (45g)	29%	32%	20%	20%

PERSONAL CONCERNS

I am not comfortable caring for residents who will die because *they* are refusing life-sustaining treatment. (35)

AGREE	DISAGREE	DON'T KNOW
17%	72%	11%

I am not comfortable caring for residents who will die because *their health care agents* refuse life-sustaining treatment. (36)

AGREE	DISAGREE	DON'T KNOW
21%	63%	15%

Appendix D
The Ethics Education Evaluation Form

ETHICS EDUCATION EVALUATION FORM

Please circle the number which best describes how you feel about each of the following questions.

1. Do you feel that you personally needed these sessions?

NOT AT ALL		SOME-WHAT		VERY MUCH
1	2	3	4	5

2. Do you feel that other nursing assistants in the group needed the sessions?

NOT AT ALL		SOME-WHAT		VERY MUCH
1	2	3	4	5

3. Do you think the sessions were interesting?

NOT AT ALL		SOME-WHAT		VERY MUCH
1	2	3	4	5

4. Do you feel that you learned anything new in the sessions?

NOT AT ALL		SOME-WHAT		VERY MUCH
1	2	3	4	5

5. Did you feel that you could speak openly about your feelings towards the different topics discussed during the sessions?

NOT AT ALL		SOME-WHAT		VERY MUCH
1	2	3	4	5

6. Do you think that participating in these sessions will help you in your job?

NOT AT ALL		SOME- WHAT		VERY MUCH
1	2	3	4	5

7. Would you recommend this ethics education program to other nursing assistants?

NOT AT ALL		SOME- WHAT		VERY MUCH
1	2	3	4	5

8. Would you want to go to more ethics sessions like this one in the future?

NOT AT ALL		SOME- WHAT		VERY MUCH
1	2	3	4	5

9. Was it helpful to have the opportunity to discuss these issues with other nursing assistants?

NOT AT ALL		SOME- WHAT		VERY MUCH
1	2	3	4	5

10. Did you like hearing what other nursing assistants had to say about these issues?

NOT AT ALL		SOME- WHAT		VERY MUCH
1	2	3	4	5

....

What did you like most about the sessions? _____
_____
_____

What did you like least about the sessions? _____
_____
_____

Are there any topics that you think we should have discussed that were not discussed at all or were not discussed in enough detail? _____
_____
_____

Please write down any comments, suggestions, or complaints: _____
_____
_____

As a nursing assistant, what types of inservices or educational programs do you think would be most valuable to you? _____
_____
_____

Thank you very much for your participation in this program! It has been a pleasure working with all of you!

Appendix E
Living Will and Health Care Proxy Forms

HEALTH CARE PROXY

(1) I, _____

hereby appoint _____
(name, home address, and telephone number)

_____

as my health care agent to make any and all health care decisions for me, except to the extent that I state otherwise. This proxy shall take effect when and if I become unable to make my own health care decisions.

(2) Optional instructions: I direct my agent to make health care decisions in accord with my wishes and limitations as stated below, or as he or she otherwise knows, or when my wishes are not clear, as my agent believes to be in my best interest. (Attach additional pages if necessary.)

Unless your agent knows your wishes about artificial nutrition and hydration (nourishment and water by a feeding tube), your agent will not be allowed to make decisions about artificial nutrition and hydration.

❏ My wishes and limitations regarding artificial nutrition and hydration are stated below:
_____
_____
_____

❏ My wishes and limitations regarding other treatments are stated below:
_____
_____
_____

(3) Name of alternate agent if the person I appoint above is unable, unwilling or unavailable to act as my health care agent.

_____

(name, home address, and telephone number)

_____

(4) Unless I revoke it, this proxy shall remain in effect indefinitely, or until the date or conditions stated below. I hereby revoke all previous health care proxies I may have executed. This proxy shall expire (specific date or conditions if desired): _____

(5) Signature _____ Date _____

Address _____

Statement by witness (must be 18 or older)

I declare that the person who signed (or asked another to sign for him or her) this document is personally known to me and appears to be of sound mind and acting of his or her own free will. He or she signed (or asked another to sign for him or her) this document in my presence.

Witness 1 _____

Address _____

Witness 2 _____

Address _____

LIVING WILL

I, _____, being of sound mind make this statement as a directive to be followed if I become permanently unable to participate in decisions regarding my medical care. These instructions reflect my firm and settled commitment to decline medical treatment under the circumstances indicated below:

I direct my attending physician to withhold or withdraw treatment that serves only to prolong the process of my dying, if I should be in an incurable or irreversible mental or physical condition with no reasonable expectation of recovery.

These instructions apply if 1) I am in a terminal condition; 2) I am permanently unconscious; or 3) if I am conscious but have irreversible brain damage and will never regain the ability to make decisions and express my wishes.

I direct that treatment be limited to measures to keep me comfortable and to relieve pain, including any pain that might occur by withholding or withdrawing treatment.

While I understand that I am not legally required to be specific about future treatments, if I am in the condition(s) described above I feel especially strong about the following forms of treatment:

I do not want cardiac resuscitation.
I do not want mechanical respiration.
I do not want a feeding tube.
I do not want antibiotics.

I do want maximum pain relief.

Other directions _____
_____
_____

These directions express my legal right to refuse treatment. I intend my instructions to be carried out, unless I have rescinded them in a new writing or by clearly indicating that I have changed my mind.

Signed: _____ Date: _____

Witness: _____

Address: _____

Witness: _____

Address: _____

Appendix F
The CNA's Ethics Booklet

FOR THE CERTIFIED NURSING ASSISTANT (CNA)

INTRODUCTION

This program looks at some of the difficult situations you may come across when you are caring for dying residents. In particular, it deals with ethical matters and treatment choices that may be made at the end of life. For example, sometimes residents choose not to have a feeding tube when they can no longer swallow, even though they know they will most likely die without the feeding tube. Cases like these and topics such as patient autonomy, living wills and health care proxies (also called the durable power of attorney for health care), truth-telling, and comfort care will be discussed during this program.

This program was developed because of two areas of interest. The first is the growing support in the United States for greater patient autonomy. (Patient autonomy is the right of the patient to make treatment decisions and to have those decisions respected and followed.) In the past, doctors used to have more control over a patient's treatment plan. It was common for doctors to be the main people who made decisions for their patients. The doctor would often make decisions about what the patient should know or not know and what types of treatment the patient should receive. Recently, however, there has been an emphasis on patient autonomy. Patients can still choose to leave their treatment in the hands of the doctor, or on the other hand, they might say, "Look, wait a minute. Tell me about my illness and my treatment choices and I'll decide what type of treatment is best for me. The doctor has the medical knowledge but he doesn't know my lifestyle, my values, my religious beliefs, and my history. Therefore, he may not be able to choose what is best for me." There are laws now that say that individuals have the right to make their own treatment choices, and patients and residents now have a legal right to decide whether they want to accept or refuse treatment. As you probably know from your own work as a CNA, in some cases patients choose to refuse treatment.

Many hospitals and nursing homes have developed ethics education programs for doctors, nurses, and social workers to teach them about patient autonomy and end-of-life ethical decision-making. Few facilities, however, have provided ethics education programs for their certified nursing assistants, the staff members who actually spend the greatest amount of time with the residents. This brings us to our second area of interest: the nursing assistant. In the nursing home, it is the nursing assistant who spends the most time with residents, gets to know residents the best, takes care of the residents' daily needs, and builds the closest relationship with residents. Sometimes the bond between the resident and CNA is family-like. Thus, when a resident dies or has chosen not to continue aggressive medical treatment (for example, refuses a feeding tube or refuses to have an amputation), it can be very difficult for all staff, but especially for the CNAs. For these reasons we thought it was important to develop an ethics education program for CNAs.

Because of your important role in caring for residents you (the CNA) should be aware of the ethical issues in end-of-life decision-making. You should know why and how certain treatment decisions are made (e.g., stopping a feeding tube or an IV), and you should know about the important positive care that you can still provide to residents even if they have chosen not to continue life-sustaining treatment.

This program will cover many issues you may come across when caring for dying elderly residents. During the educational sessions you will have the opportunity to discuss how you feel about these issues and what it's like for you in general to care for elderly residents. This project was originally carried out with over 600 CNAs from 28 nursing homes in New York and New Jersey. Some of the thoughts and feelings of the CNAs who took part in the original study are included in the instructor's manual and will be discussed during the sessions so that you can hear how other CNAs feel about these same issues. The purpose of this pamphlet is to give you a summary of some of the key points that are covered during the sessions.

PATIENT AUTONOMY

The Patient Self Determination Act (1991)

In 1991 the Patient Self Determination Act went into effect. It states that all hospitals and nursing homes that receive payments from Medicare and/or Medicaid have to tell patients and residents about their treatment decision-making rights. Basically, residents and patients have the right to know about their illness, what treatments are available to them, and about advance directives (living wills and health care proxies or durable powers of attorney for health care).

Patients and residents have the right to either accept or refuse treatment. This means that residents do have the legal right to refuse treatments such as a feeding tube, dialysis, a respirator, any medications, an amputation, etc. Residents can refuse these treatments even if it means they will die without them.

- The purpose of the Patient Self Determination Act is to place the treatment decision-making power in the hands of the patient or resident.

ADVANCE DIRECTIVES

Advance directives are written instructions of a person's treatment wishes. Advance directives are needed and used when a person can no longer make decisions or is not able to communicate his or her treatment wishes to the health care team. The two types of advance directives discussed below are health care proxies (also called the durable power of attorney for health care) and living wills. Advance directives are useful for everybody, not just nursing home residents or hospital patients.

1. *Health Care Proxy (Also Called the Durable Power of Attorney for Health Care)*

- The health care proxy is a legal document in most states. It is a form in which you write down who you want to make treatment decisions for you if there ever came a time when you could no longer make decisions for yourself.
- The person that you name in the health care proxy to make treatment decisions for you is called your *health care agent.*
- The health care proxy gives your health care agent only the ability to make health care decisions for you. (For example, your health care agent could decide whether or not you should have an amputation if you had gangrene, but *could not* make financial decisions for you.) The health care agent is not responsible for paying for your health care treatment.
- The health care proxy form must be filled out while you still have the ability to make decisions. Your family cannot decide who your agent should be if you can no longer make decisions on your own. Therefore, once a person has lost the ability to make decisions, a health care agent can no longer be chosen. Keep in mind that a person is often able to choose who she would want to make treatment decisions for her even after she has lost the ability to make more complicated decisions.
- You can always change your instructions in your health care proxy form. Just tear up the form and make a new one. If more than one form exists the most recent form will be used.
- When you choose your health care agent you should choose the person you most trust to make health care decisions for you. You should talk to your health care agent about your treatment wishes so that he/she will be able to carry out your wishes if you can no longer make your wishes known.
- If you can still make decisions on your own the doctor must ask *you* about the type of treatment you want, not your health care agent. You still have the authority to make decisions (you can ask your family or friends for their opinions but you are still the most important decision-maker). Your health care agent can only make decisions for you once you lose the ability to make decisions.
- The purpose of the health care proxy is to ensure that your treatment wishes are carried out even when you can no longer communicate those wishes to the health care team.
- If you are caring for a resident who has a health care agent and the health care agent is now making decisions for the resident because the resident cannot make decisions for herself, keep in mind that the resident chose that person to be her agent. He or she is the person that the resident wants and trusts to make health care decisions. Even if the health care agent lives in another city or doesn't come to visit that often, he or she is still the person that *the resident chose* to make treatment decisions.
- The health care agent can accept a treatment for the resident (for example, she can sign permission for an amputation), as well as refuse treatment for the resident (for

example, she could instruct the doctor not to amputate because she believes that the resident would not want the amputation).

2. *Living Will*

- The living will is a document in which you write down the type of medical treatment (antibiotics, feeding tubes, amputations, pain medications, etc.) that you would want or not want under different conditions.
- The living will must be completed by you while you are still able to make decisions.
- You can change the instructions in your living will at any time. You can just tear up the living will and start over. If there is more than one living will the most recent one will be used.
- Living wills that state things like "I do not want any *heroic measures*" are not useful because it is unclear what is meant by the words "heroic measures." If you complete a living will it should state exactly the type of treatment you would want or not want (respirator, feeding tube, IVs, pain medication, etc.).
- The purpose of the living will is to make sure that your treatment wishes are known and carried out even if you can no longer communicate those wishes to the health care team.

To Sum Up

A health care proxy or durable power of attorney for health care allows you to choose someone to make health care decisions for you if there ever comes a time when you cannot make decisions on your own. In a living will you actually write down the types of treatment you would want or not want.

The nursing home has a legal obligation to respect the wishes of the health care agent and the instructions written in a living will.

TRUTH-TELLING

Residents have a right to know about their medical condition. The amount of information a person wants to know about their own condition will depend on the person. The health care staff should try to find out what kind and how much information the resident wants to know, and then give them that information. For example, if a resident is having tests to find out what is wrong with him, the doctor should tell the resident that he is doing the tests and should ask the resident how much he wants to know about the results; for example, whether he would want to be told if they find a serious, life-threatening condition, or would prefer not to be told that kind of information and just let the doctor handle it however he thinks best.

COMFORT CARE

For many nursing home residents comfort care is just as important if not more important than aggressive medical treatment, and it is the CNAs who provide most of the hands-on comfort care.

As with all types of treatment, people feel differently about how they want their pain to be treated. Some peoples' main concern is to stop any discomfort or pain even if that means they need to be sedated. Some want quality time with friends and family and therefore may want some pain medication but not enough to put them to sleep. Others want to continue aggressive treatment in the hopes of finding a cure, even if that means their pain will increase. One of the roles of the health care team is to determine the residents' comfort care wishes and try to carry them out to the best of their abilities.

Barriers to Comfort Care

It is possible to prevent most (though not all) dying residents from feeling much pain. However, even though it is possible to prevent dying residents from feeling much pain, residents often do not get satisfactory pain relief. There are a number of things which may prevent residents from getting adequate pain relief:

- **Fear of hastening death**—Health care staff are often scared that too much pain medication will make the resident die sooner. However, staff often underestimate the amount of pain medication that residents can take, and it is rare that pain medication will "cause" death. The person may die soon after receiving pain medication, but it is the illness that is responsible for the death—not the pain medication.
- **Fear of the patient or resident becoming addicted to the pain medication**—Very few patients actually become addicted to pain medication; and in a dying resident does it really matter if the resident becomes addicted to the medication? The focus of care should be on keeping the resident as comfortable as possible.
- **Belief the patient does not really need the medication**—Sometimes staff think the resident does not really need pain medication. They think the pain is "in the resident's head" or they just want attention. The resident or patient is the best judge of their own pain. If they say they are in pain, they most likely are.
- **Not enough attention paid to signs of discomfort**—This is especially important in nursing homes where many of the residents have dementia and cannot tell the staff they are in pain. Studies have found that patients who are unable to communicate receive less pain medication than patients who can communicate and have a similar illness.
- **The resident's reluctance to increase their pain medication**—Residents sometimes don't want to take too much pain medication because they have wrong information about the medication or illness. The resident might think that if they take too much pain medication now the pain medication will no longer work on them later. Residents might also think that the pain is an expected part of their illness and there is nothing that can be done about it. Additionally, residents often feel that they don't want to "bother" the health care staff about their pain.
- **Misunderstanding the resident's wishes**—A resident who requests not to continue aggressive medical treatment is not asking for an end to all treatment. The resident still needs and wants to have comfort care. In fact, when the resident is dying he or she is especially in need of comfort care.

- **Fear of being with a dying residents**—Many people fear death and it can be difficult for people, even health care workers who frequently come into contact with the dying, to be alone in a room with someone who is near death.

The CNA's Role in Comfort Care

While medications are often used for pain relief, there are a wide range of comfort measures that are just as important in relieving pain and discomfort and that are provided by CNAs. These include:

- **Positioning**—At its most basic, positioning is needed for good circulation and to prevent skin breakdown. However, positioning also includes things like placing a resident's favorite blanket or pillow next to them, or placing their favorite picture where they can see it, or knowing the resident likes to sit five feet from the nurses station and placing the resident there.
- **Hygiene**—It is a given that residents should always be kept clean as well as comfortable. As in the case with positioning, extra touches can be provided. In our facility some of the CNAs call this "beauty care." This includes: braiding the resident's hair, applying makeup, and generally caring for the outward appearance of the resident. This can make the resident feel better about him or herself, and even if the resident is unaware of how he/she looks this increases the human contact between the resident and CNA. Additionally, it may make the family feel better to see this kind of comfort and attention given to the resident.
- **Cold compresses**—Along with medication, cold compresses can be effectively used to reduce fever and soothe the resident.
- **Mouth care**—Mouth care has been found to be an extremely important part of comfort care. While older residents who are dying often cannot tell us (because of dementia or stroke) what makes them uncomfortable, studies have been done with cancer patients to find out what are sources of discomfort. Cancer patients who were no longer taking food or water by mouth or by feeding tube/IV said they did not feel hungry but felt very uncomfortable because their mouths were so dry. This discomfort due to thirst or dry mouth can be relieved with the use of ice chips or swabs (McCann, Hall, & Groth-Junker, 1994). Dry mouth can be very uncomfortable for residents and good mouth care makes them feel much better.
- **Touch**—Just holding the resident's hand or brushing the resident's hair lets the resident know there is someone nearby who cares.
- **Talking to residents**—Many residents have few visitors and are lonely. Having someone pay attention and talk to them can be soothing to residents. Even if residents can no longer understand and respond, the sound of a familiar voice still gives comfort.
- **Paying attention to the resident's condition**—You (the CNA) spend more time with residents than any other member of the health care team. As a result, you are more likely than other people to sense changes in the resident's comfort level. Any changes in the resident's appearance, movements, breathing, or sounds that the resident makes such as moaning may be indications of pain.

Spiritual Care

One type of comfort care is spiritual care. In addition to the care provided by clergy, spiritual care can be thought of as any type of compassionate care that respects the religion and dignity of the resident. Thus, spiritual care can be provided by all staff. Spiritual care can include things like:

- sitting in a room with a dying resident
- giving comfort to a resident who is scared
- holding the resident's hand
- caring for the resident's body after death

While it is important to provide comfort and spiritual care, staff should be careful not to impose their own religious views on a resident.

STAFF SUPPORT

As you well know, in nursing homes CNAs often care for the same residents for months or even years. Because of this, when a resident dies it can be very difficult for the CNAs. CNAs we spoke to in the original study said that when some of their residents died it was like losing a family member or a close friend.

CNAs and other staff members have not always been given support when a resident dies. There has often been a feeling that "this is a professional relationship and you should not get too close to the resident." While it may help some people to try and maintain their distance from the residents, most staff say it is impossible not to care about the residents they work with. Additionally, they feel it is good for the residents to have a CNA who cares about them. Therefore people are starting to recognize that CNAs and other staff members need greater support when the residents they are working with are dying or have died. Unfortunately, support programs for nursing home staff are only developing slowly. There are a few things that you can do for yourself and the other CNAs you work with:

- Be aware that it may be emotionally difficult for you when a resident dies even if you didn't think you were that close to the resident.
- Know that you did what you could for the resident. Keeping a resident comfortable, especially when he or she is dying, is probably one of the most important things you could ever do for someone.
- If you have a case that you find very difficult, try to find someone to talk to about it, for example a fellow CNA, the nurse on your unit, a staff development person, or the nursing director.
- Be supportive of other CNAs who have lost a resident they are close to.

CONCLUSION

Slowly, around the country, people are starting to recognize that CNAs play one of the most crucial roles in the nursing home. We hope that the information you get from the program and this booklet will help you with the important tasks that you are faced with in your job caring for elderly nursing home residents.

REFERENCES

Beauchamp, T. L., & Childress, J. F. (1989). *Principles of biomedical ethics.* New York: Oxford University Press.

Buckman, R. (1992). *How to break bad news: A guide for health care professionals.* Baltimore: The Johns Hopkins University Press.

The Hastings Center. (1987). *Guidelines on the termination of life-sustaining treatment and the care of the dying.* Indianapolis: Indiana University Press.

McCann, R. M., Hall, W. J., & Groth-Juncker, A. (1994). Comfort care for terminally ill patients: The appropriate use of nutrition and hydration. *Journal of the American Medical Association, 272*(16), 1263–1266.

Morrison, R. S., & Siu, A. L. (1998, May). *Inadequate treatment of pain in hip fracture patients.* Paper presented at the meeting of the American Geriatric Society, Seattle, Washington.

Pellegrino, E. D. (1992). Is truth telling to the patient a cultural artifact? *Journal of the American Medical Association, 268*(13), 1734–1735.

Solomon, M. Z., O'Donnell, L., Jennings, B., Guilfoy, V., Wolf, S. M., Nolan, K., Jackson, R., Koch-Weiser, D., & Donnelley, S. (1993). Decisions near the end of life: Professional views on life-sustaining treatment. *American Journal of Public Health, 83,* 14–25.

Wilson, S. A., & Daley, B. J. (1998). Attachment/detachment: Forces influencing care of the dying in long-term care. *Journal of Palliative Medicine, 1,* 21–34.

Springer Publishing Company

Geriatric Nursing Protocols for Best Practice

Ivo Abraham, PhD, RN, FAAN, **Melissa M. Bottrell,** MPH,
Terry Fulmer, PhD, RN, FAAN, and
Mathy D. Mezey, EdD, RN, FAAN, Editors

"The book will be helpful to practicing nurses, to students in advanced geriatric practice, to families, and to administrators. It should be strongly recommended and widely read."

-Claire M. Fagin, PhD, RN

"I believe this is a significant contribution to the field of geriatric care and destined to become a classic."

–Pricilla Ebersole, PhD, RN, FAAN
Editor, Geriatric Nursing

The fourteen clinical protocols in this book address key clinical conditions and circumstances likely to be encountered by a hospital nurse caring for older adults. They represent "best practices" for acute care of the elderly as developed by nursing experts working with the Hartford Foundation's Nurses Improving Care to the Hospitalized Elderly project (NICHE). The protocols reflect both current research in geriatric care and a prototype for nationally promulgated nursing standards. Although the protocols were developed for acute care, they can be easily modified to work in other practice settings, such as the nursing home or home care.

Contents: Assessment of Function • Sleep Disturbances in Elderly Patients • Eating & Feeding Difficulties for Older Persons • Urinary Incontinence in Older Adults • Assessing Cognitive Function • Acute Confusion/Delirium: Strategies for Assessing and Treating • Preventing Falls in Acute Care • Preventing Pressure Ulcers • Depression in Elderly Patients • Ensuring Medication Safety • Pain Management • Use of Physical Restraints in the Hospital Setting • Advance Directives: Nurses Helping to Protect Patients' Rights • Discharge Planning and Home Follow-up of Elders • Implementing Clinical Practice Protocols

1999   256pp.   0-8261-1251-X   hard   www.springerpub.com

536 Broadway, New York, NY 10012-3955 • (212) 431-4370 • Fax (212) 941-7842

S *Springer Publishing Company*

Nursing Home Federal Requirements and Federal Guidelines to Surveyors, 4th Edition

James E. Allen, PhD, MSPH, CNHA

In a highly accessible and user-friendly format, Allen presents the latest federal guidelines and procedures that federal surveyors implement to certify facilities for Medicare and Medicaid. This updated edition contains information essential for nursing home administrators, as well as educators and professionals preparing for licensure.

New and expanded topics in the fourth edition include federal regulations on drug use and medication. These policies incorporate a quality assurance program which the Federal Health Care Financing Administration mandates for nursing facilities. Administrators who implement these regulations will have outstanding risk management and quality assurance programs in place.

For nursing home administrators, health administrators, and graduate level gerontology students.

Includes:

- Table of Contents by Federal Tag Numbers
- Table of Contents by Subject
- Federal Requirements and Guidelines
- Survey Procedures for Long-Term Care Facilities
- Index

2000   440pp.   0-8261-8123-X   soft   www.springerpub.com

536 Broadway, New York, NY 10012-3955 • (212) 431-4370 • Fax (212) 941-7842